The Infertility Journey

The Infertility Journey

Real voices. Real issues. Real insights.

Tarun Jain MD

www.theinfertilityjourney.com

Medical disclaimer:

This book is intended to be a guide and not a prescription for your health issues. The ideas, suggestions, and procedures contained in this book are not intended to be a substitute for consulting with a qualified health care professional. All matters regarding your individual health require personal medical supervision. Neither the author nor the publisher shall be liable or responsible for any loss or damage allegedly arising from any information or suggestion in this book.

Clomiphene (Clomid), Letrazole (Femara), Norethindrone (Aygestin), Medroxyprogesterone (Provera), Metformin (Glucophage), Leuprolide (Lupron), Ganirelix, Antagon, Gonal-F, Follistim, Bravelle, Menopur, and Ovidrel are registered trademarks.

ISBN-13: 9781535129169
ISBN-10: 1535129166
Library of Congress Control Number: 2016906298
CreateSpace Independent Publishing Platform
North Charleston, South Carolina

Acknowledgements

*"As we express our gratitude, we must never forget that
the highest appreciation is not to utter words, but to
live by them."*
- John F. Kennedy

SPECIAL AND SINCERE thanks to all the patients, doctors, nurses, advocates, and artists who contributed in some way to this book.

To my dear wife Ruchi,

our parents, our friends, and our children Rohan & Riya.

Table of Contents

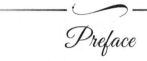

Preface

"Everything will be okay in the end. If it's not okay,
it's not the end."
- John Lennon

INFERTILITY N. "THE inability to conceive a child."

Subfertility n. "The inability to conceive a child after a certain time period; Lower fertility than a typical couple."

- Infertility is the commonly used term that often encompasses the term 'subfertility'.
- Medical criteria:
  - woman under 35 has not conceived after 12 months of contraceptive-free intercourse.
  - woman over 35 has not conceived after 6 months of contraceptive-free intercourse.
- Infertility affects approximately 15 percent of couples (1 in 7) in the United States.
- Primary infertility – woman has never been able to conceive to date.
- Secondary infertility – difficulty conceiving after having previously conceived.

- Women become less fertile as they get older. The impact of age on male fertility is less clear.
- Infertility occurs equally among women and men. About 35% of infertility is related to the male partner, 35% to the female, 20% involving both partners, and the remaining 10% being unexplained.

Introduction

*"One of the most valuable things we can do to heal one another
is listen to each other's stories."*
- Rebecca Falls

THERE ARE MANY things in life that we often take for granted. One of them is the ability to have children. Most people don't expect to have difficulty having a child. We have thought about it, and have a vision in our minds of when and how it will all happen. We want to plan it out, so it fits in with our life timeline. However, when things don't go as planned … the infertility journey begins … and is often one of the most difficult and trying times in your life.

The infertility journey, however, does not have to be so difficult. By being empowered with the right information, you can make the right choices … leading to the most efficient path to success. It is with this goal in mind, that I decided to write this book. I want everyone who is dealing with infertility to have the relevant medical information at his or her fingertips.

I also want you to know that you are not alone. Your story is not that different than millions of other couples facing infertility. We are all human and have similar emotions and feelings. Having treated hundreds of couples, I realize that most are all going through the same emotions, struggles and pitfalls. The same questions and dilemmas of what to do. The same social stigmas and feelings of isolation, blame, and guilt.

I therefore wanted to keep this book simple yet powerful. I included the most pertinent medical information that is also easy to understand. I also added numerous cartoon depictions of positive and negative comments that couples with infertility often encounter. I further included anonymous quotes from many infertility patients to put real voices behind the disease. You should know that what you are feeling is real and shared by many others.

Keep this book next to you as you go through your journey. You may also want to share it with close family and friends. It will help them better understand your struggle.

Finally, know that there is light at the end of your journey. Most every person who has patience and persistence goes on to have a successful outcome. The road may get bumpy, but keep the faith. It is all worth it in the end … which of course, is the start of a new beginning!

Warm wishes,
Tarun Jain, MD

Part One

The Basics

FAMILIES-TO-BE
By Bonniejean Alford

This journey unplanned, seemingly unwanted,
yet ever accepted as the path necessary
for an unknown final destination that awaits.
Continuity of faith builds a love undeniable,
even as anger builds toward the heavens.
Peace permeates heart and soul,
despite the reality that biology seems to have failed;
Creation evidently needs a helping hand.
Here, now, science blesses the bodies
in which lay the future of legacies:
Families-to-be very much in waiting.
Hope rests in the hands of those chosen to protect,
surviving in the training that has prepared them to assist
along this most unexpected and important journey,
no matter the final destination.

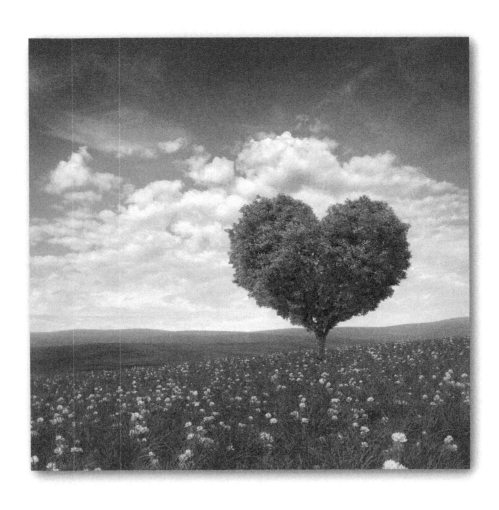

CHAPTER 1

—

Trying To Conceive

"Don't wait for the perfect moment. Take the moment and make it perfect."
- Zoey Sayward

CONCEPTION. A PROCESS that is often taken for granted. It is frequently expected to happen whenever a couple is ready to have a child. It is sometimes even planned in such a way that a couple can time the ideal birthday for their anticipated child. Contraception is often extended in order to allow for careers to be built and finances to be put in place.

After all, if so many other couples have children, getting pregnant must be a pretty quick and easy process ... right?

Let's begin with the process of conception. How does a pregnancy occur?

1. The ovary must develop and release (ovulate) a healthy egg (oocyte).
2. This single, microscopic cell must be captured by the fallopian tube within a few hours before it disintegrates.
3. Ejaculated sperm must travel from the vagina, past the cervical canal / mucus, into the uterus, and thru the fallopian tube to meet the egg. Out of millions of sperm deposited, only a few hundred make it to the egg.
4. Sperm can survive within the female reproductive tract for up to 3 days.
5. Fertilization (successful joining of egg and sperm) must occur within the fallopian tube.

6. The fertilized egg (embryo) must travel thru the fallopian tube and enter the uterus.
7. The embryo must continue to develop and grow normally.
8. The developing embryo must successfully implant into the lining of the uterus (endometrium).
9. Pregnancy! The cells of the early pregnancy produce a hormone called human chorionic gonadotropin (hCG) that is detected via a blood or urine test.

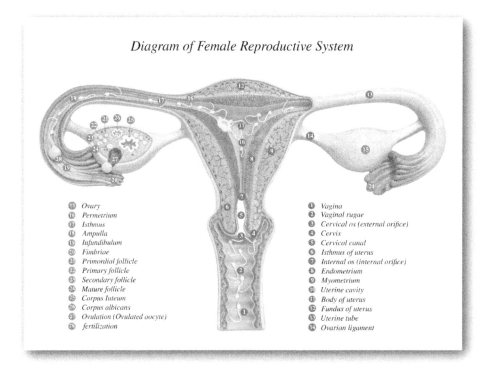

Diagram of Female Reproductive System

⑮	Ovary	❶	Vagina
⑯	Permetrium	❷	Vaginal rugae
⑰	Isthmus	❸	Cervical os (external orifice)
⑱	Ampulla	❹	Cervix
⑲	Infundibulum	❺	Cervical canal
⑳	Fimbriae	❻	Isthmus of uterus
㉑	Primordial follicle	❼	Internal os (internal orifice)
㉒	Primary follicle	❽	Endometrium
㉓	Secondary follicle	❾	Myometrium
㉔	Mature follicle	❿	Uterine cavity
㉕	Corpus luteum	⓫	Body of uterus
㉖	Corpus albicans	⓬	Fundus of uterus
㉗	Ovulation (Ovulated oocyte)	⓭	Uterine tube
㉘	fertilization	⓮	Ovarian ligament

Given the timing, coordination, and complexity of all these steps, it is therefore not unusual for conception to take some time for any couple. About 85% of young healthy couples should get pregnant within a year, and 92% within two years. Women over age 35 and men over age 50 have lower fertility rates. A biological problem within any of the above steps is unfortunately common and can lead to infertility.

Trying To Conceive

Tips

1. Before attempting pregnancy, make sure you adopt a healthy lifestyle and take prenatal vitamins. Folic acid in prenatal vitamins reduces the risk for major birth defects.
2. Fertility is decreased in women who are very thin or obese. Aim for an ideal body weight (BMI 19 - 25).
3. If you have a known medical or genetic condition, seek advice from your doctor before getting pregnant.
4. The 'fertile window' is the time in a menstrual cycle when pregnancy can occur. It is a six-day interval that begins five days prior to ovulation and ends on the day of ovulation.
5. The highest chance of pregnancy occurs with intercourse every 1 to 2 days during the fertile window.
6. Urinary ovulation predictor kits are an effective means to detect the day of ovulation. However, false-positive results occur in about 7% of cycles.
7. Sexual position, orgasm, or prolonged rest after intercourse does not increase the chance of conception.
8. Avoid lubricants such as K-Y® Jelly, K-Y® Touch, Astroglide®, saliva or olive oil which can have a negative impact on sperm quality. Safer lubricants include Pre-Seed®, canola oil or mineral oil.
9. The following lifestyle factors have a negative impact on fertility:
   - Smoking and alcohol consumption (more than 2 drinks per day) in both men and women.
   - Caffeine (more than 200mg per day or 3 regular cups of coffee per day) is associated with subfertility and higher miscarriage rates.
   - Illicit drugs (marijuana) and exposure to toxic substances (such as agricultural pesticides and radioactivity).
   - Prolonged exposure to high heat (saunas, steam rooms, hot tubs) can lower sperm quality.

Quotes

"I am just really starting to face the reality that we may not have children. I did not realize how long we had been trying until I thought about our 5-year anniversary coming up. I tried not to worry about getting pregnant. Now I feel like time is running out."

•••

"My husband and I have been TTC (trying to conceive) for about a year and we're not getting anywhere. I have never had a regular period so I was already mentally prepared to see a fertility doctor."

•••

"I am a step mom. My husband has kids from a previous relationship and he is an excellent dad. I often feel sad sometimes because I just hope that soon we will be able to have our own together. I LOVE my step kids to pieces and they love me too, but I just want to have my own so I can be called 'mommy'."

•••

"When I see people in social settings with their kids, I dream of introducing them to my own child instead of hearing them say 'You don't have any kids yet?' And, with a smile I reply 'Nope not yet' crying on the inside ready to quickly change the subject. And somehow they always slip in and ask 'Why... don't you want kids?' My response is always the same, 'Of course but it just hasn't happened yet.'"

•••

"I never expected to have to deal with infertility at such a young age but now that I am a bit older and ready to start a family I feel a bit lost about how to go forward with getting my hopes up to high."

• • •

"It's frustrating and annoying when there are others around you who are pregnant."

• • •

"Sometimes I just wonder why this life is so unfair. I just don't know how much of this infertility I can handle. I wonder why God does this sometimes, and why he makes us struggle so. I just feel like I am never going to be able to have children."

• • •

"My husband and I have been desperately trying to conceive for about 8 months. I know that's probably not very long compared to how long other people have been trying, but I'm worried because I have one son (7 years old) and I had no issues conceiving him. We haven't been to a doctor about it yet, but I'm beginning to get very worried and have been extremely depressed. It seems like all my friends can get pregnant with the drop of a hat and I hate to admit it, but I feel a bit envious ... I feel very bad for feeling that way."

• • •

"Bottom line is that this has been a frustrating road and I never wanted our intimacy to become a chore - which it really has. I hate constantly thinking about what time of the month it is - if timing is right - if position is right - if we shouldn't use lubricant because it kills sperm - and everything else I've read online. Then thinking every little pinch or twinge means that we conceived. I'm kind of driving myself crazy - and its taking away from the experience that I always envisioned of a baby just happening - I know it's naive to think. I hate to say it but I don't look forward to sex anymore because it seems so mechanical - a means to an end."

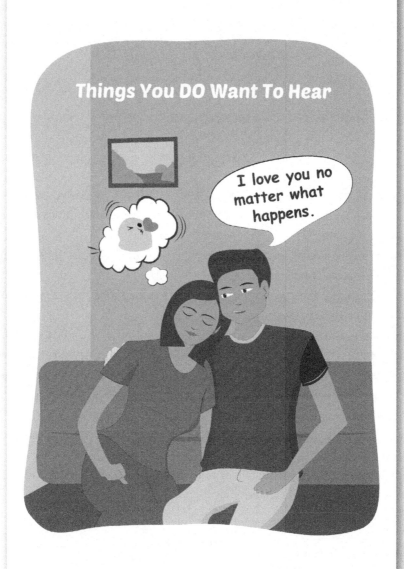

C H A P T E R   2

Diagnosis Of Infertility

*"Failure will never overtake me if my determination to succeed
is strong enough."*
- Og Mandino

INFERTILITY -- A disease, defined as the inability to achieve a successful pregnancy after 12 months or more of regular unprotected intercourse (or 6 months if over age 35).

Infertility is common. Approximately 1 out of 7 couples in the United States has trouble conceiving.

Couples who have been trying to conceive for more than a year should seek an infertility evaluation. For women who are 35 years or older, you should begin an infertility evaluation after six months of unprotected intercourse. However, if you have a known or suspected infertility-associated condition (such as PCOS or endometriosis), you should seek assistance earlier.

The range of emotions that arise from the inability to have a child are vast and powerful. Some common feelings may include sadness, frustration, anger, guilt and jealousy. It can also have a negative impact on the relationship between couples.

Infertility is an equal opportunity disease. In other words, the cause can equally originate from the female or male (and often both). The following is a general breakdown of the causes:

i. Female Factors:

- Ovulatory issues – hormonal imbalances can frequently disrupt this complex process; often due to Polycystic Ovary Syndrome (PCOS).

- Endometriosis – tissue that normally lines the inner uterine cavity (endometrium) is present outside the uterus (commonly on the outer surface of the ovaries, fallopian tubes, and uterus).
- Tubal disease – blockage/damage within or around one or both fallopian tubes; commonly due to past infections.
- Uterine disease – the presence of fibroids, polyps, or scar tissue within the uterine cavity can hinder sperm transport or embryo implantation.
- Advanced ovarian age – increase in female age from about 27 onwards leads to a progressive decline in egg number/quality and hence fertility. This fertility decline becomes steeper after age 35.

ii. *Male Factors:*

- Sperm quality – decreased volume, concentration, motility, and/or morphology (shape/size of sperm).
- Erectile dysfunction – difficulty initiating or maintain an erection.
- Undescended testis – present from birth.
- Scrotal varicocele – enlarged scrotal blood vessels (veins) that alter testicular temperature and blood flow.
- Ejaculatory problem

iii. *Unexplained*

- No obvious cause identified after an infertility workup.
- Abnormalities may be present but not detected by current methods.
- Possible problems include:
  - Poor egg quality
  - Egg not released at optimal time
  - Egg not entering the fallopian tube
  - Sperm not reaching the egg
  - Fertilization failure
  - Problem with transportation of fertilized egg into uterus

o   Poor embryo development
o   Implantation failure

Tips

1. Regardless of the diagnosis, most couples have success with fertility treatments.
2. Do not underestimate the negative impact of advancing female age on fertility.
3. Seek help early (especially if you are over 35 years of age) to avoid the increasing stress and frustrations that can come with advanced infertility.
4. It is important to know that the uterus does not change with increasing age (only the ovaries). This allows women of advanced age to conceive using younger eggs from another woman (donor eggs).

Quotes

"It's hard to concentrate on everything that you are blessed with when the infertility is so heavy on your mind."

• • •

"As I'm in my mid-30s, I'm coming to terms that one of the hardest things about infertility, is that the alternative, being child free is not well accepted. I feel that people must be looking at me and are judging that at my age, I am either infertile or selfish."

• • •

"After 7 months of perfect ovulation tracking and having sex at the 'perfect' times with no success, we started the process of figuring out our issues. One sperm analysis later, we were told that our only chances of conception was doing IVF with ICSI...period."

•••

"I hate that I can't just get pregnant like everyone else I know, but being a mom has always been a dream of mine so I'm determined to do anything possible to have a child."

CHAPTER 3

Seeing My Ob/Gyn

"He is the best physician who is the most ingenious inspirer of hope."
- Samuel Taylor Coleridge

IT IS COMMON for women with infertility to initially seek the guidance of their Obstetrician/Gynecologist (Ob/Gyn) doctor. Some Ob/Gyns have a special interest in evaluating and initially treating infertility. Other Ob/Gyns may choose to refer you to a Reproductive Endocrinologist right away (RE; aka 'fertility specialist') – discussed in the next chapter.

Ob/Gyns with experience in infertility treatment will begin with a history and physical examination. This should generally be followed by the following basic tests:

- Blood hormone testing (FSH, Estradiol, TSH, and Prolactin)
- Hysterosalpingogram (HSG) - assess your uterus and fallopian tubes
- Semen analysis (SA)

If the above tests are normal, your Ob/Gyn may recommend a 3-month trial of Clomiphene Citrate (Clomid®) with timed intercourse. Assessment of ovulation is often recommended via ovulation predictor kits (available over the counter) or by checking your progesterone blood level. A progesterone level over 3.0 ng/dl means you ovulated in your current cycle.

If you do not get pregnant after this 3-month approach, it is common for your Ob/Gyn to refer you to an RE specialist.

Seeing My Ob/Gyn

Tips

1. Be pro-active and let your Ob/Gyn know when you are planning to expand your family.
2. Ask for help early (especially if you are over 35 years old) if you are having difficulty. Female age is critical.
3. If the semen analysis is abnormal or you have blocked fallopian tubes, ask for a referral to an RE.
4. If you have a history of irregular periods (which implies ovulation problems) or endometriosis, seek help right away.

Quotes

"I remember asking my Ob/Gyn if it was okay for me and my husband to try and conceive even at my weight and she said "of course" and said she did not see a problem with it at all. She said that since I had regular monthly cycles all should be fine."

• • •

"You don't have to start with an RE, you can go to your Ob/Gyn for starters. If you are older than 35, go now because you don't want to waste any time."

• • •

"I would personally start with an RE and go from there. I think lots of time, money, and emotional energy is often wasted with OB/Gyns, who simply are not infertility experts."

• • •

"Knowing what I know now, I would not wait more than a year before seeking help, and I would not have wasted more than a couple cycles of testing with my OB before going straight to an RE. You can have some tests done with an OB, but they are not experts on getting pregnant, they are there for all that comes after."

• • •

"I am 28 years old and my husband and I have been trying for almost two years. We are currently seeing my Ob/Gyn and all the tests came back good. My struggle now is all the people around me who are getting pregnant ... like my sister in law and people I work with. I am discouraged to the point where I don't want to even exercise anymore because I keep hoping I will get pregnant. Every month I experience 'symptoms' of early pregnancy and chalk it up to thinking about it so much. Everyone I talk to tells me to stop trying so hard but how do you do that?!"

• • •

"If you get a Doc that gives you a prescription and tells you to watch for an LH surge with these strips you buy at the store or just hopes you get lucky, then I recommend you find a new Doc as this Doc is wasting your time, emotion, and money."

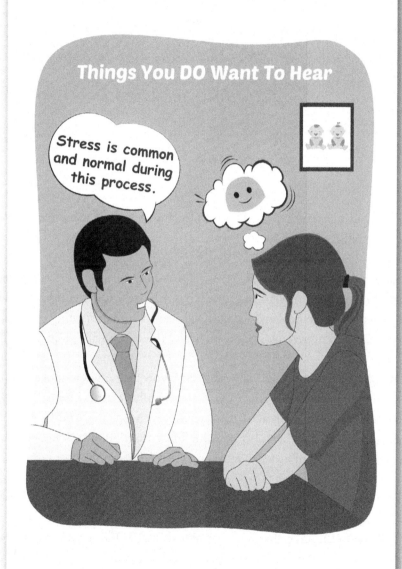

CHAPTER 4

Referral To Reproductive Endocrinologist (Fertility Specialist)

"Once you choose HOPE, anything is possible."
- Christopher Reeve

THE NAMING TERMINOLOGY can be confusing. Here are some basic definitions to be familiar with:

Reproductive Endocrinologist (RE) – also known as a 'fertility specialist'; a specialized Ob/Gyn physician who, after completing the full 4-year Ob/Gyn residency training, has completed 3 additional years of formal training (fellowship) in Reproductive Endocrinology and Infertility (REI) at an approved program.

ABOG (American Board of Obstetrics & Gynecology; www.abog.org) – an independent non-profit organization that annually certifies about 1,700 Ob/Gyns and subspecialists in REI, Maternal-Fetal Medicine, and Gynecologic Oncology in the US. They also examine more than 30,000 Board-Certified physicians each year in order to maintain their certification status.

Board Certification in Obstetrics & Gynecology – This is the first Certification achieved by an RE after passing a rigorous written and oral examination in Ob/Gyn that is administered by ABOG. It demonstrates that the doctor has competence in the latest medical guidelines, treatments, and techniques in general women's health care.

Referral To Reproductive Endocrinologist (Fertility Specialist)

FACOG (Fellow of The American Congress of Obstetricians and Gynecologists) – also referred to as an 'ACOG Fellow'. It is a special certification given only to doctors who are Board Certified in Ob/Gyn. It demonstrates additional competence and peer recognition in general Ob/Gyn care.

Board Certification in Reproductive Endocrinology & Infertility – This is the highest certification achievable by an RE. An RE who is 'Board Certified in Reproductive Endocrinology & Infertility' has not only passed Board Certification in Ob/Gyn, but has also passed additional rigorous written *and* oral examinations by ABOG specific to REI topics. It demonstrates that your doctor has demonstrated special knowledge and professional qualifications related to Infertility, and has competence in the latest fertility treatments.

ASRM (American Society for Reproductive Medicine; www.asrm.org) – a non-profit organization that provides information, education, advocacy and standards in the field of reproductive medicine. ASRM also publishes 'Fertility & Sterility' which is the leading peer-reviewed medical journal dedicated to infertility. Most RE's are members of ASRM, regardless of their certification status.

SART (Society for Assisted Reproductive Technology; www.sart.org) – an affiliated society to ASRM. It is dedicated to the practice of IVF and represents the more than 90% of the IVF clinics in the country. The mission of SART is to establish and maintain standards for ART so that you receive the highest possible level of care. SART also collects and publishes IVF pregnancy and birth outcome data from its member clinics.

While some infertility couples initially seek the care of their Ob/Gyn, some will go directly to an RE in their area. Regardless of your choice, it is vital for you to find a physician whom you feel comfortable with and trust.

There are several ways to find a qualified RE:

- Ob/Gyn referral
- Internet search engine
- Word of mouth (family, friend)
- Insurance company referral
- ASRM or SART Websites

Both you and your partner/spouse should attend the first meeting together. Infertility is a shared experience that will require mutual understanding and support. The first meeting is often enlightening, educational, and even emotional. You doctor will know the sensitive and stressful nature of your visit. Since over 25% of couples have more than one cause of their infertility, it is very important to talk to and evaluate both you and your partner.

The following initial tests are commonly recommended and performed by your RE (there may be others depending on individual circumstances):

1. Blood tests
   a. Cycle Day 3 FSH and Estradiol (E2) -- assess impact of age on fertility (ovarian reserve)
   b. Anti-mullerian hormone (AMH) -- assess impact of age on fertility (ovarian reserve)
   c. Thyroid stimulating hormone (TSH) -- check for an over- or under-active thyroid gland
   d. Prolactin (PRL) -- check for an overactive pituitary gland
   e. Progesterone -- confirms if ovulation has occurred
2. Imaging studies
   a. Pelvic ultrasound -- check uterus and ovaries
   b. Hysterosalpingogram (HSG) -- check inside shape of uterus and if your fallopian tubes are open
   c. Saline infusion sonogram (SIS; sonoHSG; "water ultrasound") -- check if uterine cavity is free of polyps, scar tissue and fibroids

  d. Office Hysteroscopy – office procedure to directly visualize the uterine cavity

Tips

1. Plan early to see an RE. It can often take 2-4 months from the time an appointment is made till all of your testing is completed.
2. Prior to your visit, write your questions and concerns on a piece of paper to make sure they all get addressed and answered.
3. Create an 'infertility journey diary' to keep yourself organized.
4. The topics covered can be overwhelming and complex. Feel free to ask your doctor and nurse questions whenever you need clarification.
5. Good news: you will find that fertility treatments offer more hope than ever before. Most patients who seek care from an RE reach their goal of having a baby.
6. Trust your instincts – if you don't feel comfortable with a specific doctor, don't hesitate to get another opinion.

Quotes

"I spent a long time trying with a regular Doc and then switched after about 1 1/2 years of trying to an RE."

•••

"DONT WAIT!!! That is my best advice. Even if you come out of the RE's office with a 'bad' diagnosis, that wouldn't change if you waited a year or two longer out of fear. It would possibly make it worse."

•••

"Nobody should have to tolerate a physician who isn't attentive, providing details, exhausting options, and who doesn't have appropriate bed-side manners!"

• • •

"I highly recommend an RE because their specialty is fertility and getting women pregnant as well as hormones and that is something that even the best OB/Gyns are not very good with as they just dabble in it and try this or that. Plus, usually an RE will do much more testing up front and that is a good thing because the RE can find problems and fix them or bypass them with certain types of treatment before you go spend several cycles doing things by a guess that would have never worked."

• • •

"My husband and I have been trying to conceive for 3 1/2 years without success, mostly blown off to, 'don't worry about it, you're so young', so after approximately 6 months on Clomid® and 6 months on Femara® and Metformin, we were sent to an RE."

• • •

"We were told to wait a year. But I waited 4 months and explained to my RE that we didn't wait because we knew something was wrong. You have to be proactive in this. I'm glad I didn't wait, because waiting a year would mean getting treated after about another 6 months to a year. I feel like that would be wasting time, and the clock is ticking for us. I'll be 32 soon and don't want to feel like I'm racing against my eggs age."

• • •

Referral To Reproductive Endocrinologist (Fertility Specialist)

"A few of my friends started with their Gyn and the tests weren't as extensive and they just went on Clomid® for a while and then eventually wound up with an RE."

• • •

"Success rates alone may not represent the services provided by a clinic. I've read from somewhere that a lot of clinics have their criteria of accepting patients and rejecting patients who do not meet their standards. So it might be helpful to look at the statistics in the context of how many and who their patients are."

• • •

"We tried for over 2 years with just tracking ovulation. If I had gone to a RE way back then I would have known not to waste those 2 years because it will never happen for us naturally. Now my eggs are 2-plus years older."

• • •

"Never lose your hope! It's good that we have a fertility specialist now to help us. We are one huge step closer to our aim. There are a lot of women whose tests come back normal when still combating the IF issue but they get pregnant with professional help."

• • •

"The trick really is to never lose hope and always have a plan for the next cycle. If you stay on the journey, then you will eventually get to your goal and a very large part of a successful journey for so many is with professional help."

• • •

"At our first appointment with an RE, I was devastated. I cried in his office. I knew we had a problem; I didn't know how bad it was. The sooner you know, the sooner you can start working towards your goal."

• • •

"After meeting with my RE, I was so happy that there was a chance. An expensive chance. but some is better than none. I understand that feeling of it being cold. It's not heartwarming to say we did it at a sterile clinical environment. But I figure if we are successful in having a baby, I can tell him when he grows up that we loved him so much that we endured so many RE visits, pokes and prods, exams, and financial hurdles just to have him. I don't think there's any shame in it. I think by having to conceive this way just shows how dedicated we are."

• • •

"I think we need to write down all of our questions as we think of them so we won't forget during the consultation."

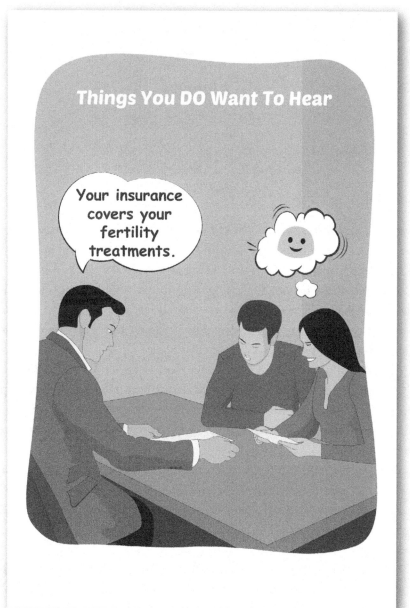

CHAPTER 5

Finances

"What I know is that if you do work that you love, and the work fulfills you, the rest will come."
- Oprah Winfrey

FINANCIAL CONSIDERATIONS IMPACT nearly all couples. The costs of raising a family are daunting enough. Dealing with potential medical costs related to fertility treatment will certainly bring added challenges and stress.

To begin with, do not make any assumptions. Most importantly, don't assume fertility treatment will be too expensive and not worth pursuing. Costs and coverage can vary widely. Furthermore, less than 3% of infertile couples need the more expensive IVF treatment.

Many employers provide insurance with fertility benefits. There are also several states that have laws (mandates) requiring employers to provide fertility benefits. The states currently with the best fertility mandates include Massachusetts, Illinois, New Jersey, Connecticut, and Rhode Island.

Be proactive and call your insurance carrier to determine your fertility benefits. Most fertility centers will also help determine what fertility services are covered by your insurance. Specific questions to ask your health insurance provider include:

- What is the definition of infertility in order to qualify for coverage?
- Do I have coverage for fertility testing? If so, what testing is covered (bloodwork, HSG, sonoHSG, semen analysis)?
- Do I have coverage for fertility treatment? If so, what treatments are covered (Intrauterine insemination? In vitro fertilization?)

Finances

- Do I have coverage for fertility medications? If so, which medications (Clomid®, Letrazole, Follicle Stimulating Hormone, Progesterone, GnRH agonist, GnRH antagonist)?
- What are my deductibles and co-pays?
- Do I need a referral?
- Are there any restrictions on which fertility specialist I can see?

Even if the coverage is not what you were hoping for, do setup an initial consultation to learn your options. Many fertility centers have opportunities to finance your treatment (similar to financing for a car or home). Furthermore, it may be likely that you will not need the advanced and more expensive treatments.

Tips

1. Bottom line – Don't shut the door on the dreams of having a child based solely on financial concerns.
2. If your insurance company denies coverage, ask them about their appeal process.
3. Several fertility medication manufacturers provide discounts to patients based on financial need.
4. Talk to your human resources (HR) department at work to learn about different insurance coverage options. Keep track of when your open enrollment period occurs each year, in case you need to make health insurance changes.
5. Many programs provide discounts if you are in the Military.

Quotes

"I would LOVE to do fertility testing but unfortunately our insurance does not cover it."

•••

"I have insurance that covers everything except for PGD and its unlimited coverage. And, so far they are wonderful!!!!"

•••

"My insurance policy covers up to $25,000 in fertility treatment but only $5,000 in meds (I used that up my first cycle). Unfortunately, I found out yesterday that they won't cover anything for donor eggs which is what I will be now doing as well."

•••

"My insurance pays nothing until I meet my deductible and even then only pays for the diagnostic workup for infertility and no infertility treatments or meds."

•••

"My insurance is military and only pays for diagnostic testing and covers cycles using timed intercourse only. If I were to have added an IUI or done IVF, then it no longer covers anything and we were quoted $15,000-$18,000 for an IVF cycle with ICSI. We ended up getting into an IVF program for military at a reduced cost, thank God, because otherwise we would not have been able to afford it."

•••

"I hope it works because I have had to save the money for this procedure and for medication. My insurance covers NOTHING!! My husband is the only one working so everything falls on him. I am a full-time student and was considering a part-time job but my husband wants me to focus on school."

•••

"I think men just want us to be happy and hate to see us hurting so badly. And then they try to wrap their brain around why things cost so darn much. I told my husband a million times, we are not paying for the treatments, we are investing in our future child."

•••

"My husband is so practical and I say cold...no feelings go with his decisions. It's a practical reasoning because of finances for him. And for me, if I could do it tomorrow I'd find a way."

•••

"Just be aware that mandated coverage may NOT mean they will cover IVF. The mandate varies by state."

•••

"We are all out of money and I am willing to take a job anywhere to get infertility coverage."

Part Two

The Causes

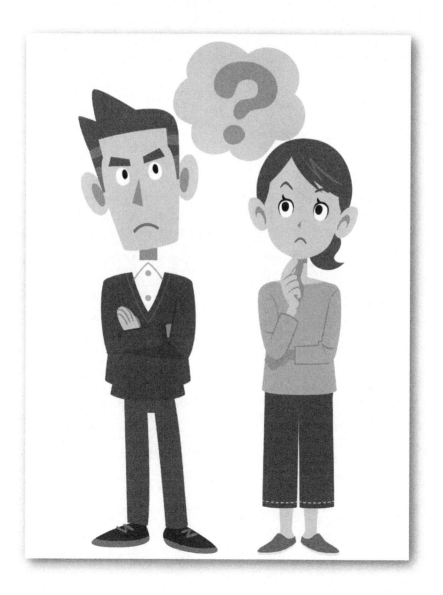

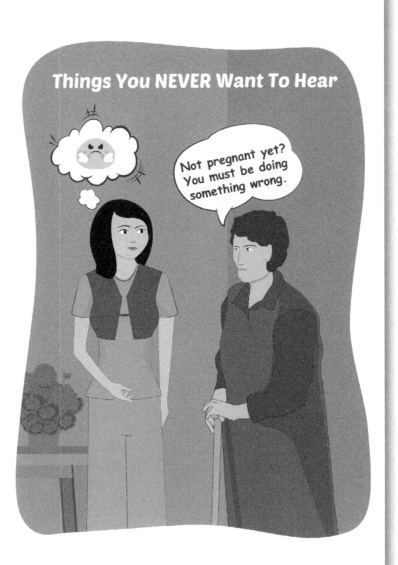

CHAPTER 6

Polycystic Ovary Syndrome (PCOS)

*"If you are always trying to be normal, you will never know
how amazing you can be."*
- Maya Angelou

POLYCYSTIC OVARY SYNDROME (PCOS) is a common hormone disorder that affects 5-10% of *all* women.

There are a lot of misconceptions about how PCOS is diagnosed. The diagnosis involves a woman meeting 2 of the following 3 criteria:

1. Chronic lack of ovulation (infrequent or absent menstrual cycles)
2. High testosterone blood level or increased body hair growth/acne
3. Ultrasound demonstrating ovaries with multiple small follicles (cysts)

Besides infertility due to lack of ovulation, women with PCOS are also at risk for the following:

1. Metabolic syndrome — obesity, high cholesterol, high blood pressure, and insulin resistance/diabetes. These symptoms can subsequently increase the risk of heart disease.
2. Endometrial cancer — when ovulation does not occur, estrogen from the ovaries continues to stimulate the lining of the uterus (endometrium). If this continues over a long period of time, the endometrium may begin to undergo precancerous changes. It is therefore important

for women with PCOS to not go without having a period for more than 4-6 months.

If a woman is overweight/obese, weight loss can help improve ovulation patterns and fertility. Even 5-10% weight loss can be beneficial. Insulin-sensitizing medicines such as metformin can help improve ovulation and also lower the risk of developing diabetes or metabolic syndrome.

There are several fertility methods available to help induce ovulation for women with PCOS. Common first-line oral medications include Clomiphene (Clomid®) or Letrazole (Femara®). If unsuccessful, injected fertility medications called gonadotropins may be given to stimulate the ovaries. IVF is also considered if other treatments are not successful.

Women with PCOS undergoing fertility treatment must be carefully monitored due to an often-unpredictable response to medications. Responses can vary from being slow at times, while other times being high with too many follicles/eggs developing. A high response can lead to an increase in risk of multiple births or ovarian hyperstimulation syndrome (OHSS).

If fertility is not the goal, the following various treatments may help correct PCOS symptoms:

1. Oral contraceptive pills (OCP; the pill) – can regulate menses, reduce extra hair growth/acne, and lower risk of endometrial cancer
2. Metformin - can decrease the risk of developing diabetes or metabolic syndrome
3. Spironolactone – can lower male hormones to treat excess hair growth and acne
4. Mechanical hair removal – via electrolysis and laser treatment
5. Weight loss – via diet modification and exercise

Treatments will be individualized by your doctor based on your unique needs and circumstances.

Polycystic Ovary Syndrome (PCOS)

Tips

1. Your Anti-Mullerian Hormone (AMH) level will often be elevated if you have PCOS.
2. Weight loss really helps. Ask your primary care doctor for a referral to see a nutritionist.
3. Get a pedometer to track your daily activity/steps. Try to achieve 10,000 steps a day.
4. Don't go more than 4-6 months without a period. It increases the risk of developing endometrial cancer.
5. Seek fertility help early if you know you have PCOS. You do not have to wait a full year of trying on your own.

Quotes

"I do not seem to show signs of PCOS, (not an apple shape, regular periods, sugar is not high, etc.) but I often wonder if I have it. I do have a dark patch of skin on the back of my neck."

• • •

"I am just recently diagnosed with PCOS, waiting for my primary doctor to refer me to the Ob/Gyn here in town to start meds. I had one miscarriage in February of this year and have ovulated once since then, and I am now on day 70 without a sign of the big O. I also have high LH and testosterone to boot. I am having a hard time with this, full of emotion and feeling so unsexy."

• • •

"I was finally diagnosed with PCOS in January when I was referred to an RE. I say 'finally' because I have battled with regular Ob/Gyns for about five years who have insisted that I am fine. I've had many of the signs, the hair that seems to pop up in new places daily (ahhhh), no periods unless I am on birth control pills, anovulation, & weight gain."

• • •

"I was diagnosed with PCOS at age 19 and until last month I have been on the pill ever since. Fortunately, my history of PCOS was well documented so my Ob/Gyn is pursuing treatment a bit more aggressively than others might. She had me do a couple cycles off the pill just testing for ovulation, and since that yielded nothing we are going to start Clomid® with my next cycle. I hope it will do the trick."

• • •

"I was dx with PCOS last April. My husband I have been going to an RE since December. Right now I am on Metformin and have tried 3 IUIs with no luck. We are going to try this month on our own and if that doesn't work we are going to get more aggressive with the meds. We are hoping to start our family soon. It is so hard to be around people who are able to get pregnant so easily. Our best friend happens to be some of those people, they tried for 3 months and she just delivered her baby yesterday."

• • •

"I have never had a normal period. It happens about once a year without birth control pills or Provera. The docs always said I was too skinny (not anymore) and probably exercised too much (Ha!) and basically brushed me off with the word, 'it's not a big deal until you try to get pregnant.' So here I am at the age of 30 and married and you guessed it trying to get pregnant. What a pain!"

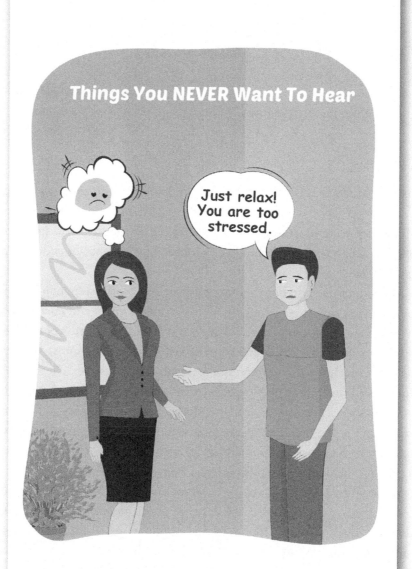

CHAPTER 7

Endometriosis

"When you can't change the direction of the wind – adjust your sails."
- H. Jackson Brown Jr.

ENDOMETRIOSIS IS COMMON and occurs in 3-10% of women of reproductive age, and 25-50% of women with infertility. It is defined by the presence of tissue from the uterine lining (endometrium) outside of the uterus (most commonly on the ovaries and behind the uterus). The presence of endometriosis can ultimately lead to pain and infertility.

Many theories exist, but the exact cause of endometriosis remains unclear. The most common theory suggests that in some women, endometrial tissue flows through their fallopian tubes and implants in other areas of the pelvis.

Many women with endometriosis have few or no symptoms. Some may experience severe menstrual cramps, painful intercourse, or chronic pelvic pain. Other women may only experience infertility.

Symptoms may be suggestive of endometriosis, but surgery (typically via laparoscopy) is the best way to diagnose endometriosis. Ultrasound may be helpful in the diagnosis if a woman has an endometrioma (a blood-filled ovarian cyst from endometriosis, also called a "chocolate cyst").

Surgery can not only diagnose endometriosis, but can treat it (via burning or removing the endometriosis lesions). Based on the surgical findings, endometriosis is often classified into one of four stages (I-minimal, II-mild, III-moderate, and IV-severe). The classification however does not correlate with the presence or severity of symptoms.

There is presently no cure for endometriosis. The recurrence rate after surgery is 10% within 1 year and 20% within 5 years.

Endometriosis

Endometriosis may cause infertility via creating scar tissue, blocking tubes, or releasing factors that may be toxic to eggs and sperm. Infertility patients with untreated mild endometriosis conceive at a rate of 2-4% per month (15-20% being normal). Patients with moderate to severe endometriosis conceive at less than 2% per month.

Medical treatment (via hormonal medications like birth control pills and Lupron) may control pain, but will not improve fertility. Surgical treatment has been shown in several studies to improve both pain symptoms and fertility.

Tips

1. Avoid multiple surgeries for endometriosis-associated pain unless medical management is unsuccessful.
2. Avoid surgical removal of endometriosis ovarian cysts (endometriomas) if fertility is desired, since such surgeries may reduce your ovarian reserve.
3. Medical management of endometriosis does not improve fertility.

Quotes

"I ended up having to have my fallopian tubes removed recently due to damage from endometriosis I didn't know I had. Now we are facing the shock of spending our life savings to get pregnant. I go from anger to self-pity to hopefulness just about every day."

• • •

"I have horrible endometriosis! It spread to other organs and used to squeeze them and I'd be in terrible pain. I'm a teacher and I missed the second day of school two years ago due to taking pain pills of a friend because I was desperate! They made me sick and I had to leave school after vomiting."

• • •

"I'm 27, don't have kids, and have never been able to get pregnant. My husband and I have been trying for years. We have been seeing an infertility specialist for just over a year now, and my diagnosis was always labeled as 'unknown infertility,' as all my tests always came back 'normal'. I tried Clomid®, Femara®, IUI, and even 'natural fertility' remedies at home. Nothing ever worked. Given my painful periods, my RE suggested surgery. Sure enough, my doctor found endometriosis, but she said it was only a small amount on the back of my uterus and spots on both of my ovaries. Thankfully, she was able to remove it all! I am still in disbelief and shock that I finally have a diagnosis after all this time. My periods are better now. I'm so excited and hopeful for our future."

CHAPTER 8

Tubal Disease

*"The man who moves a mountain begins by carrying away
small stones."*
- Confucius

THE FALLOPIAN TUBES are attached to the uterus on the left and right sides, and normally pick up an egg as it is released (ovulation) from the ovary. The egg and sperm meet and join (fertilize) within the fallopian tube. The fertilized egg (embryo) then travels from the tube into the uterus, where it can start attaching to the lining of the inner uterine surface (endometrium).

A blockage of one or both fallopian tubes is an important and common cause of infertility. The blockage can occur anywhere within the tubes. A blockage where the tube is attached to the uterus is called 'proximal obstruction'. A blockage at the end of the tube that picks up the egg is called 'distal obstruction'.

Pelvic infections are a common cause of tubal infertility, with many women not being aware of such damage. Most women do not have any symptoms other than fertility problems. Tubal blockages can also occur due to scar tissue from endometriosis or prior abdominal surgery.

Any woman with infertility should strongly consider undergoing a hysterosalpingography (HSG) test to evaluate her tubes. It is an X-ray test that can be performed by a gynecologist, radiologist, or fertility specialist. The doctor will inject a special liquid in the uterus that shows up on x-ray. The test will show if the liquid freely flows through the tubes, or if there is a proximal or distal obstruction. It will also show if there is a 'hydrosalpinx' – a tube that is swollen and filled with fluid due to distal obstruction.

Surgery can be considered to repair distally blocked tubes, but success is usually worse than IVF treatment. Surgery is however recommended if a woman has hydrosalpinx, since the fluid within the tubes reduces IVF success by about 50%. Surgically blocking/cutting the swollen tube or removing the entire tube (salpingectomy) from its connection to the uterus will significantly improve IVF success.

Tips

1. Many fertility doctors perform HSGs in their office – which can provide added convenience and comfort for you.
2. Fertility is often improved for a few months after your HSG (if your tubes are found to be open).
3. Taking an analgesic (like Ibuprofen or Acetaminophen) an hour before your HSG can reduce discomfort from the HSG.
4. Ask your doctor about taking an antibiotic (Doxycycline) before the HSG to reduce any infection risk.

Quotes

"I had a hydrosalpinx blocking my right tube. Had a laparoscopy last July to get it clamped. During the surgery, my surgeon also had to separate my left ovary from my uterus, as peritonitis secondary to appedicitis when I was 10 had created all this damage! I am now 18 weeks pregnant. Having a hydrosalpinx is scary, and I haven't found many others with this condition. But if your other tube is clear, you can still get pregnant naturally after the affected tube is clamped (the fluid from the hydrosalpinx is toxic to embryos). Good luck, and there is hope!"

•••

"I am 31 and both tubes are blocked (hydros). I now have a surgery date with my RE. We were originally going to remove the tubes completely, but have now decided to clamp them. This makes me feel somewhat better, as I am just not ready to get rid of my useless tubes!"

•••

"I have endometriosis - unknown stage. I went on to have two ectopics, with the second resulting in loss of my tube due to rupture. I did two rounds of IVF, with the second resulting in boy/boy twins. We are extremely grateful and blessed."

•••

"I have never been pregnant and was recently diagnosed with blocked fallopian tubes (confirmed with laparoscopy) after trying to conceive for almost 2 years. My RE told us that our best option would be IVF. My insurance does not cover IVF. It will however cover 'surgeries to correct tubal defects.' I know my chances are better with IVF, but we just can't get the money together. I feel like my time clock is clicking and I need to do something before it's too late. So, I am considering exploring the tubal surgery option."

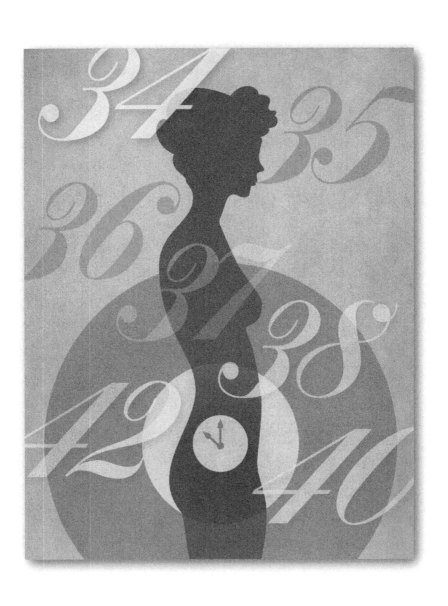

CHAPTER 9

Age Factor / Decreased Ovarian Reserve

*"Our greatest weakness lies in giving up. The most certain way
to succeed is always to try just one more time."*
- Thomas A. Edison

BASED ON UNITED States Census Bureau data, there has been an increasing trend towards delaying childbearing. The average age when couples get married has been steadily increasing along with the average age when couples have their first child. The unfortunate consequence of such a delay is that with increasing female age, there is a progressive decline in fertility.

Women are born with all the eggs (oocytes) they will ever have. At birth there are about one million eggs, which reduce to about 300,000 by puberty. Between puberty and menopause, about 300 eggs may ovulate, while the rest will undergo spontaneous degeneration. There is presently no known method to reduce the rate of egg loss. Use of birth control pills does not slow this process down, either.

Given this progressive rate of egg loss, a woman's reproductive peak occurs in her mid-upper 20's. Fertility subsequently declines in the 30's, with a steeper decline occurring after age 35. By the early 40's the chance of conception is very low. On average, an average 30-year-old woman has a 20% chance of pregnancy each month. This drops to less than 5% for a 40-year-old woman. Very few spontaneous or non-donor egg-assisted live births have been reported after age 45.

The declining quantity of eggs in the ovaries with age is also known as 'decreasing ovarian reserve (DOR)'. It is also known that the chromosomal quality of eggs decreases with age. This can lead to an increasing risk of genetic abnormalities (*aneuploidy*) and miscarriages with increasing age. At time of fertilization, an egg and sperm should each have 23 chromosomes. After fertilization, the fertilized egg (embryo) should have 46 chromosomes. Due to age related errors, the resulting embryo may often have 45 or 47 chromosomes. This is called aneuploidy and can result in no pregnancy, miscarriages, or birth defects. A commonly known aneuploidy is Down Syndrome, which results from a 47-chromosome embryo which has an extra chromosome #21 (Trisomy 21).

There are screening tests for ovarian reserve, but none have the ability to reliably predict the possibility of getting pregnant or having a live birth. A 'normal' result from these tests does not necessarily mean your ovarian reserve is normal. These tests include the following:

1. Blood FSH and Estradiol (E2) levels on day 2, 3, or 4 of your cycle
   o Day 3 FSH>10 mIU/mL and/or Day 3 Estradiol>80 pg/mL indicates decreased reserve
2. Blood Anti-Mullerian Hormone (AMH) level
   o Can be performed at any time in your cycle
   o AMH<0.5 ng/mL predicts decreased reserve with<3 follicles in an IVF cycle
   o AMH<1.0 ng/mL predicts decreased reserve with limited eggs at IVF retrieval
   o AMH>1.0 ng/mL but<3.5 ng/mL suggests good response to ovarian stimulation
   o AMH>3.5 ng/mL predicts high response to stimulation with increased risk of ovarian hyperstimulation syndrome (OHSS).
3. Transvaginal ultrasound measurement of antral follicle numbers (Antral Follicle Count; AFC) on day 2, 3, or 4 of your cycle
   o Antral follicles are small follicles measuring 2 to 10 mm in diameter
   o A low AFC (from 4-10 total follicles) suggests poor ovarian reserve
   o Less predictive of egg quality, ability to get pregnant, or pregnancy outcome

Age Factor / Decreased Ovarian Reserve

Tips

1. Ovarian reserve testing results may fluctuate if repeated. However, once a test is found to be abnormal, future results in the 'normal' range are not reassuring.
2. A younger woman with decreased ovarian reserve testing has a better prognosis than an older woman with the same result.
3. Age is still a powerful predictor of ovarian reserve. Advanced age with 'normal' ovarian reserve testing is not reassuring.
4. Current evidence suggests that AMH may be the best initial screening test for ovarian reserve.
5. Results from ovarian reserve testing should not stop you from undergoing fertility treatment.

Quotes

"I was diagnosed with diminished ovarian reserve at the age of 36. I have a child who is almost three and had no trouble getting pregnant with her. Anyway my FSH was 11.5 and I had 8 antral follicles. My RE recommended being aggressive and doing IVF. Well, after my second IVF cycle, I am so excited to be pregnant!"

•••

"I'm devastated to learn that my AMH level is 0.025! I have spent days and nights crying myself to sleep, because I know what this number means. And, going through it all alone doesn't help either. I'm 40, and facing the fact that I could never have a biological baby of my own hurts too much. I am still going to try."

•••

The Causes

"At my age (41) I've been told it's a numbers game. I can keep cycling and will eventually get that golden egg. I am at a crossroads. Even assuming infinite financial resources, the emotional and physical toll is substantial. Throw in the added pressure of advanced maternal age and it's a pressure cooker."

CHAPTER 10

Uterine Factor

"The only real failure in life is the failure to try."
- Unknown

ABNORMALITIES OF THE uterus can certainly play a role in lowering the chance of a successful pregnancy. The hypothesis is that any significant irregularity within the uterine cavity can either mechanically interfere with implantation, or prevent normal endometrial development.

The following uterine cavity conditions have been implicated with lower rates of fertility and live birth:

- Submucous fibroids (the type that grow into the cavity)
- Congenital malformations (uterine septum)
- Endometrial polyps
- Intrauterine synechiae / adhesions (scar tissue)
- Infection (chronic endometritis)

The following tests are performed to assess / rule out the above issues:

- Hysterosalpingogram (HSG) – very good at determining the presence of congenital malformations
- Saline infusion sonogram (sonoHSG) – ideal for picking up submucous fibroids, polyps, and scar tissue
- Office hysteroscopy – a very thin camera that can be used in the office to directly visualize the uterine cavity
- Endometrial biopsy – considered if infection is suspected

Fortunately, if any of the above issues are discovered, the following treatments are available and effective:

- Hysteroscopy (operative) – a simple out-patient surgical procedure where a thin instrument with a camera is inserted in the uterus via the cervix. It allows for true diagnosis and surgical treatment of fibroids, polyps, or scar tissue in the uterine cavity. It can also be used to remove a uterine septum and therefore lower the chance of a future miscarriage. The recovery time from a hysteroscopy procedure is quick (typically less than 24 hours) with minimal discomfort.
- Antibiotics – although chronic infections within the uterus are uncommon, if encountered, it can be treated with a 10-14 day course of a broad-spectrum oral antibiotic.

Note that although abnormalities with the cervix (Cervical Factor) have been described and implicated with infertility, there is no good test to assess the impact. Traditionally, the postcoital test (PCT) had been used to identify abnormalities in the quality or quantity of cervical mucous production. This test however has been well studied and found to be unreliable and not predictive of pregnancy. Do inform your doctor if you have had any procedure done on your cervix (cerclage, LEEP, cryotherapy). Such procedures may indicate potential issues with cervical weakening, narrowing, or scar formation.

Tips

1. If you have had several unsuccessful IVF cycles, consider re-assessing the uterine cavity for polyps.
2. Ask your fertility doctor about doing a sonoHSG at the same time you have an HSG done. A sonoHSG is better at evaluating the uterine cavity.
3. If you had a recent miscarriage, consider doing a sonoHSG or office hysteroscopy to make sure the uterine cavity is clear.

4. Spotting in the middle of your cycle can be an indicator of polyps.
5. Heavy or long-lasting periods can be an indicator of submucous fibroids.

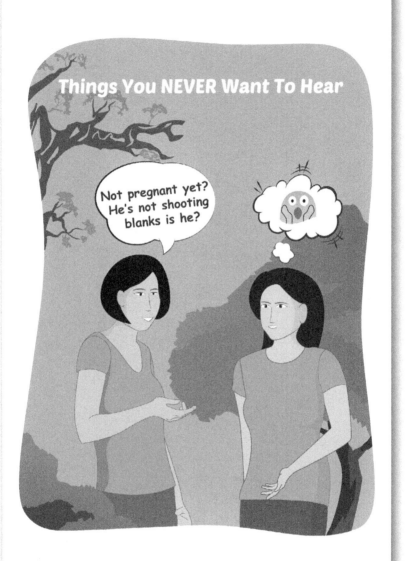

CHAPTER 11

Male Factor

"It's hard to beat a person who never gives up."
- Babe Ruth

MALE FACTOR IS common and is found in about 35% of all couples presenting with infertility.

The initial testing involves at least one semen analysis. Most commonly, the man masturbates into a sterile plastic cup that is provided by the doctor's office or andrology laboratory (a lab that specializes in dealing with male fertility). The semen can be collected at home, provided the specimen can be delivered to the testing center in less than an hour after ejaculation. Many fertility centers have designated rooms for men to produce the semen in a comfortable and private setting.

Sperm can also be collected during sex in a special condom provided by the doctor. If a man is suspected to have retrograde ejaculation, the sperm can be retrieved in the lab from urine he has collected. Men who have a difficult time with erection or ejaculation despite using medications, as well as men with a spinal cord injury, may be able to produce a sperm sample with the help of procedures such as vibratory stimulation or electro-ejaculation.

The important parameters of a semen analysis include the volume, concentration, motility, and morphology. Your doctor should go over these numbers with you.

- Volume: the total amount of semen in milliliters (ml)
- Concentration: the number of sperm found per milliliter of semen
- Motility: the percentage of sperm that is moving

- Morphology: the percentage of sperm that are of normal shape and size

If the initial semen analysis is abnormal, your doctor may recommend a repeat semen analysis as well as referral to a fertility specialist. Depending on the degree of abnormality, the fertility specialist may recommend blood hormone testing or possibly referral to a Urologist.

Tips

1. Ask your doctor to have a semen analysis performed before starting any fertility treatment.
2. If a semen analysis is significantly abnormal, consider repeating it.
3. If significant 'Round Cells' or White Blood Cells (WBC) are noted in the semen, this may indicate an ongoing inflammatory process that needs antibiotic treatment.
4. Smoking and marijuana use can negatively impact sperm quality.
5. Sperm takes about three months to develop and mature before ejaculation.

Quotes

"Just because you are young doesn't mean everything is fine. That is the worst advice doctors can give. My cycles were 100% normal, always on time, I still ovulate every single month, everything like a 'normal, fertile person', but if I would've been more proactive instead of waiting around for it to happen, I would have found out sooner that my hubby had 0% normal sperm."

•••

"We just found out our problem is due to my husband's low sperm count, secondary to a medication he's been on for years. My concern now is my husband's sadness over it being a 'problem' with him. He's feeling like a failure as a man and worried that, if through science, we aren't able to conceive I'll want a divorce or be disappointed in our marriage."

•••

"Although the problem with conception lied with my wife not ovulating, I was told my sperm count was extremely low. When I received the news, as I presume any man would feel, I was dejected. I believed differently. I believed if every man in my family was able to conceive, why couldn't I?"

•••

"My husband and I are dealing with male factor infertility. It's a difficult process for both parties, because, let's face it, we all look at ourselves as here to reproduce. I feel that men tend to be more emotional and harder on themselves when it is male factor. My husband has low count as well as morphology and we have been directed to do IVF since we started going to our doctor. It has taken a while for my husband to accept it, but now we are excited! I had a lot of the sympathy talks with him to lift his spirits but you can't give too much sympathy (if that doesn't sound heartless?). My husband was ashamed, I guess you could say, such that he didn't even like talking about it - especially when trying to decide our next step. But it got to the point where I had to tell him to suck it up because it's life and this is the hand we have been dealt with, and if we want kids, we need to make our next step. He has to understand that: 1) it's both of you who are dealing with this not just him and, 2) that it is extremely common for couples to have to undergo some sort or fertility treatment. No one really knows how common infertility is until you are amongst the group."

•••

"My husband researched donors while he was home recovering from his sperm extraction surgery. He felt it helped him heal emotionally and that if he couldn't contribute genetically, this was a way he could contribute to the conception process."

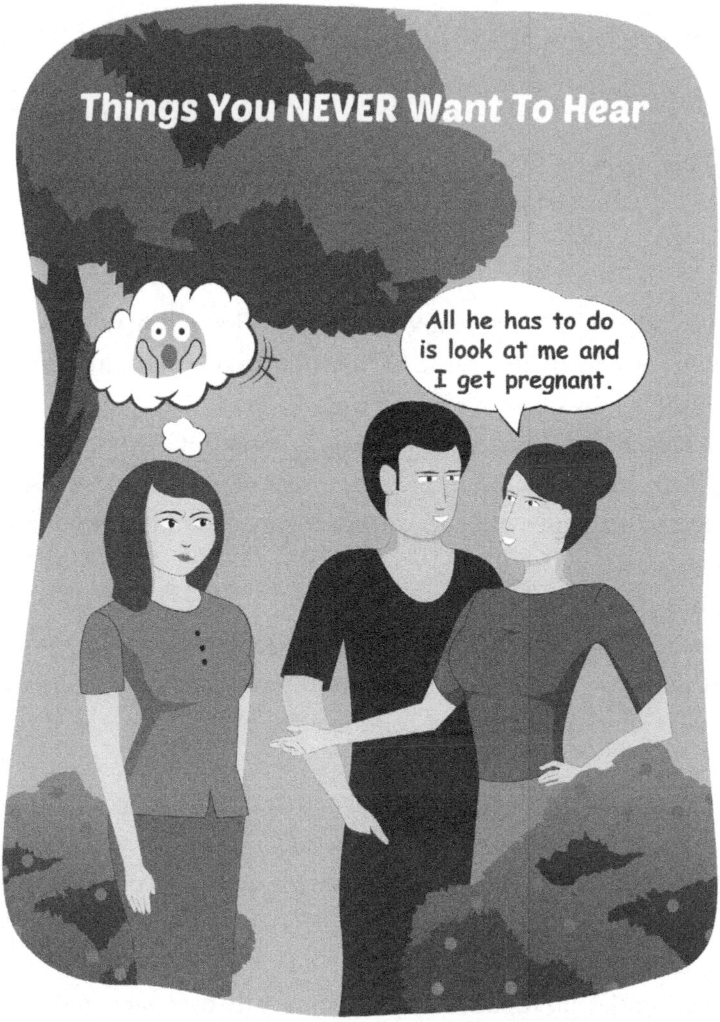
Things You NEVER Want To Hear
All he has to do is look at me and I get pregnant.

CHAPTER 12

Unexplained

"True freedom lies in the realization and calm acceptance of the fact that there may very well be no perfect answer."
-Allen Reid McGinnis

APPROXIMATELY 15-20% OF couples with infertility will have normal testing results, with no identifiable cause of infertility. Such cases are referred to as "unexplained". This is often a frustrating diagnosis for couples since everyone is looking for an answer to the basic question of: 'why can we not get pregnant?'. In such circumstances, there may be other hidden factors that are difficult to diagnose with current technology. Examples include problems with sperm function, fertilization, egg quality, genetic factors, undiagnosed endometriosis, implantation, or tubal function.

Although it is a frustrating situation, the good news is that most couples with this diagnosis go on to conceive and have a live birth. The following options are often recommended / considered:

1. Laparoscopy – to diagnose/treat endometriosis, especially if there is a high clinical suspicion (painful periods)
2. Superovulation with IUI – treatment with oral or injectable medications to induce the ovaries to produce more than one dominant follicle
3. In vitro fertilization (IVF) – to potentially overcome 'hidden' factors related to endometriosis and sperm / egg interaction

Unexplained

Tips

1. Even with such a diagnosis, many couples achieve success with fertility medications along with timed IUI.
2. IVF has been shown to be the most effective treatment for unexplained infertility.

Quotes

"It was so frustrating to get a diagnosis of unexplained infertility after completing all the testing. We have been trying to get pregnant for four years and thought something would have come up for sure."

•••

"We have been trying for 2.5 years. We have been going to a fertility clinic and thus far, our diagnosis is unexplained. My numbers are good, and her numbers are good. All tests, bloodwork, scans, etc. are good. Of course, now my wife is depressed. Hard on herself; blaming herself for us not having a child ... I don't know what to do. I try to be happy and upbeat and supportive for her. I provide a shoulder for her to cry on."

Part Three

The Treatments

CHAPTER 13

Clomiphene Citrate (Clomid®)

*"There are two primary choices in life; to accept conditions as
they exist, or accept the responsibility for changing them."*
- Denis Writley

CLOMID® IS ONE of the most widely used medications used to treat infertility. It is an oral medication that is an anti-estrogen. In simple terms, it fools the brain into thinking there is not much estrogen in the body. This evokes a response from the brain to increase production of hormones (FSH) that stimulate ovarian follicular development. It is often prescribed for patients who either do not ovulate on their own (PCOS), or for patients who do ovulate, but need an extra boost to potentially produce more than one egg.

Clomid® is typically started on either cycle day 3, 4, or 5 with a starting dose of 50mg per day for 5 days. The use of daily doses greater than 150mg or for longer than 5 days has limited efficacy. Ovulation with use of Clomid® can be spontaneous (via the body's own LH surge) or induced via injecting human chorionic gonadotropin (hCG). Proof of ovulation can be determined via a mid-luteal (approximately cycle day 21) serum progesterone level (>3 ng/ml indicates ovulation occurred).

Approximately 80% of women will respond well to Clomid®, with most requiring daily doses of 100mg or less. Side effects from Clomid® can include hot flashes, headaches, and mood changes (in about 10% of women). Rarely, visual disturbances (such as halos, blurring, or streaks around lights) can occur. The chance of twins with Clomid® is about 7% if you are pregnant (risk of triplets or more is very low).

The Treatments

Tips

1. Mood changes with Clomid® can be especially bothersome and disturbing. Let your doctor know early, so alternatives can be discussed.
2. There is no significant difference whether Clomid® is started on day 3, 4, or 5 of your cycle.
3. Higher doses of Clomid® can sometimes lead to a thinner endometrial lining, which may not be favorable.

CHAPTER 14

Aromatase Inhibitors (Letrazole & Anastrozole)

"The secret of change is to focus all of your energy, not on fighting the old, but on building the new."
- Socrates

LETRAZOLE (FEMARA®) & Anastrozole (Arimidex®) are in a class of medications called 'Aromatase Inhibitors', because of their mechanism of action. Aromatase is an enzyme in the body that helps convert testosterone to estrogen. The medication works by inhibiting the enzyme, aromatase, and thus lowering estrogen levels.

Aromatase inhibitors are presently FDA approved in the US for the treatment of breast cancer in postmenopausal women. They are however being used with increasing frequency in the US for ovarian stimulation (since about 2001). By the lowering of estrogen levels, aromatase inhibitors cause a reflex increase in pituitary production of FSH, which subsequently stimulates the ovaries.

They are prescribed for ovulation induction in a similar manner as Clomid®. Typically, the pills are taken for five days starting on cycle day 3, 4, or 5. Letrazole is more commonly prescribed, with a starting dose of 2.5mg once a day. Other doses include 5.0mg or 7.5mg once a day. Common side effects may include hot flashes, fatigue, and dizziness. The risk of multiples is low (about 3-5% chance of twins). Early studies raised concern that letrazole was associated with an increased risk of congenital abnormalities, but subsequent studies to date have not reproduced these findings.

A recent well-designed study (2014) indicates that the ovulation, pregnancy, and live birth rates with Letrazole are significantly higher than with

Clomid®, among infertile women with PCOS. This study also confirmed no significant differences in birth defect or miscarriage risk between Letrazole and Clomid®.

Tips

1. Letrazole is being used with increasing frequency as a first-line medication to treat infertility. Ask your doctor about it.
2. Letrazole is less likely to have the bothersome side effect of mood changes that may often accompany Clomid® use.

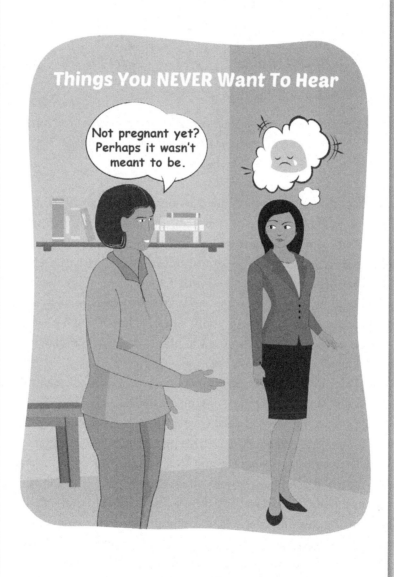

CHAPTER 15

Gonadotropins (The "Injectables")

"Everyone faces challenges in life. It's a matter of how you learn to overcome them and use them to your advantage."
- Celestine Chua

GONADOTROPINS ARE FERTILITY medications that contain FSH alone, or in combination with LH. They are not available as an oral medication, and need to be injected subcutaneously (just under the skin, typically in the low abdomen).

They are frequently used to stimulate ovarian follicular development in patients who have not had success with Clomid® or aromatase inhibitors. They may also be used as first-line medications to treat women whose pituitary gland does not make enough FSH and LH (hypothalamic amenorrhea). These same medications are also used in higher doses to stimulate the ovaries for in vitro fertilization (IVF) cycles.

Gonadotropins are considered 'stronger' than the oral medications since they can often result in the development of multiple follicles/eggs. The benefit of multiple follicles is an improved chance of pregnancy. The downside is the higher potential for multiple pregnancy or ovarian hyperstimulation syndrome (OHSS).

Most fertility centers manage non-IVF stimulation cycles in a standard manner. After a baseline ultrasound on cycle day 2 or 3, the gonadotropin is injected once daily (typical starting dose is 75 to 150 IU), over a period of 7 – 13 days. During this time, periodic ultrasounds are done to measure follicular development along with blood tests to measure estrogen levels. Depending on the monitoring results, the gonadotropin dosing can be adjusted.

The objective is often to produce one or two dominant follicles (16-20 mm in diameter), but can vary depending on your individual circumstances. Once this objective is reached, ovulation is triggered via an hCG injection. If too many follicles have developed or the estrogen level is too high, your doctor may recommend cancelling the cycle to avoid an increased risk of multiple pregnancy or OHSS.

hCG (human chorionic gonadotropin) is normally produced by the placenta, and has similar structure and function to LH. Therefore, similar to the LH surge, an hCG injection will cause a follicle to release its egg. The hCG injection is also often used to trigger ovulation when Clomid® or Letrazole are used. Keep in mind that a pregnancy test may give a false positive result if done within 10 days after administering the hCG.

Tips

1. Some injectables come in an easy-to-use pen device – ask your RE or nurse.
2. The hCG injection is equally effective via a subcutaneous or intramuscular route.
3. Severe OHSS will not develop if the hCG injection is not administered.
4. There is no clinical difference between different brands of the injectables.

Quotes

"Don't be afraid! It is really just all of the what if's that make you anxious, but if you do injections they really aren't bad and not even close to what you conjure in your mind and the IUI itself isn't bad either."

•••

"I received my box of meds this morning, it's pretty intense!! I wish someone would have told me NOT to look at the size of the needles."

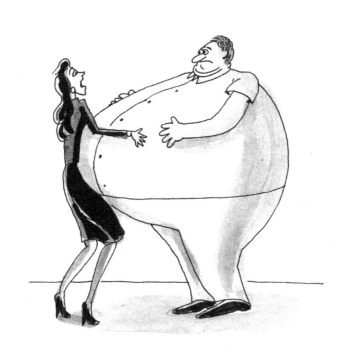

"I'm not sure this is going to work out."

CHAPTER 16

Intrauterine Insemination (IUI)

"I've learned the main thing in life is that you get what you put in."
- Adele

THE CERVIX NATURALLY limits the number of sperm that can enter the uterus. Therefore, only a few sperm actually make their way to the fallopian tubes. Intrauterine insemination (IUI) is a common office procedure that bypasses the cervix and places sperm into a woman's uterus near the time of ovulation. The goal is for the sperm to be closer to the awaiting egg, and therefore have a greater likelihood of fertilizing it.

Previously stored (frozen) or fresh sperm may be used for an IUI. The semen sample is prepared by the lab before insemination. The process involves 'washing' the sperm by removing the seminal fluid (which can otherwise cause cramping), and concentrating the viable sperm. An analysis by the lab gives a number called the 'Total Motile Count (TMC)'. For optimal outcomes, the TMC should be greater than 10 million sperm.

The IUI is typically performed 24 to 36 hours after the hCG trigger (close to the time of predicted ovulation). It is unclear if a consecutive day (double) IUI has added benefit over a single IUI.

The IUI procedure takes just a few minutes and is done in the office either by a clinician or doctor. After the woman lies on the exam table, a speculum is inserted in the vagina. A catheter is gently inserted into the uterus via the cervix. This part can sometimes be challenging depending on the curvature of the uterus. Once the catheter is in place, the washed semen sample is gently injected into the uterus, followed by removal of the catheter. There may be some cramping, but the procedure is usually painless. Sperm travels very quickly and can make it to the tube/egg within a few minutes or less.

Success from IUI depends on the cause of infertility. IUI is more effective than timed intercourse. It is recommended for couples with simple ovulatory issues, unexplained infertility, or for mild sperm quality issues. It is not recommended if a woman has tubal disease, severe endometriosis, or severe male factor.

Overall success rates can be as high as 20% per cycle depending on female age, diagnosis, and type of fertility medications used.

Tips

1. Strongly consider adding IUI to your ovulation induction treatment regimen. It will significantly improve your odds of pregnancy.
2. Many fertility centers offer the possibility of producing the semen on site (especially if you live more than an hour away).

Quotes

"I find myself disappointed that we're not able to do it 'naturally'. We want a family and look forward to raising children - and I can't help but think that conceiving a child through the route of artificial insemination is so ... cold? I can't describe it - and I think I need to reboot my thinking."

CHAPTER 17

Surgery

"The most reliable way to predict the future is to create it."
- Abraham Lincoln

NOBODY LIKES OR wants to undergo surgery. Anytime surgery comes up as an option, anxiety usually follows. If surgery is a consideration, it is important for you to determine the potential risks and benefits.

From a fertility perspective, there are a few common reasons to consider surgery. They include the following:

1. Endometrial polyps
   - Typically suspected after completing a hysterosalpingogram (HSG) or saline infusion sonogram (sonoHSG)
   - Presence may lower chance of pregnancy and/or increase risk of miscarriage
   - Recommended surgery: Hysteroscopy with polypectomy
2. Uterine fibroids
   - Common finding after ultrasound; size and locations can vary
   - Fibroids that are growing into the uterine cavity ('submucous' type) found based on HSG or sonoHSG, may lower chance of pregnancy and/or increase risk of miscarriage; may also contribute to heavy periods
   - Recommended surgery: Hysteroscopy with myomectomy

3. Intrauterine adhesions (scar tissue inside the uterus; also known as 'Asherman Syndrome')
   o   may occur due to prior infection or uterine surgery
   o   Presence may lower chance of pregnancy and/or increase risk of miscarriage
   o   Recommended surgery: Hysteroscopy with lysis of adhesions
4. Endometriosis
   o   Associated with infertility; often associated with pelvic pain
   o   Surgery is the only way to diagnose; can be concurrently treated; no cure; may recur
   o   Surgical treatment improves fertility
   o   Recommended surgery: Laparoscopy with fulguration of endometriosis (use of electrocautery or laser to burn the endometriosis areas)
   o   Special consideration: endometrioma is an ovarian cyst due to endometriosis; individual circumstances warrant surgery to remove the cyst versus leaving them alone
5. Hydrosalpinx (fluid-filled, blocked fallopian tubes)
   o   Usually picked up via HSG or pelvic ultrasound
   o   Presence will lower chance of pregnancy, even via IVF treatment
   o   Recommended surgery: Laparoscopy with removal or clamping of the affected tube(s)
6. Ovarian cyst (simple; follicular)
   o   Frequently occur and often regress on their own within one to three months
   o   Persistent cysts that are large or not regressing can delay fertility treatments
   o   Recommended surgery: Transvaginal cyst aspiration or Laparoscopic cyst removal
7. Polycystic Ovary Syndrome (PCOS)
   o   For select patients who do not respond to medical treatment
   o   Recommended surgery: Laparoscopy with ovarian drilling

Surgery

Quotes

"My doctor had me do both the saline sonogram and HSG dye test prior to starting IVF. I was glad that he did because they didn't find anything in the dye test- all my pipes were clean but in the saline test they found several polyps in my uterus. I had to have them surgically removed- an embryo would never have implanted with them there."

•••

"My HSG test didn't find polyp in uterus, but saline test did. With that polyp out of my system, I am now praying for my successful IVF."

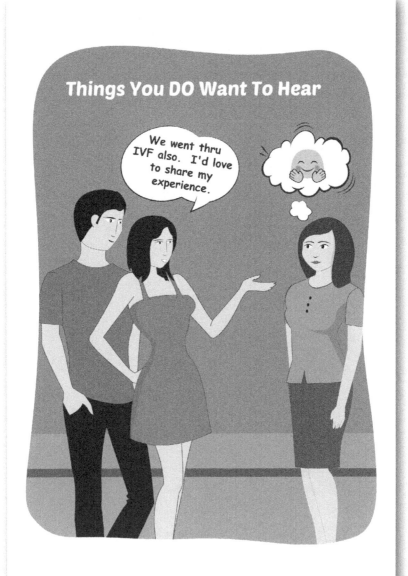

CHAPTER 18

In Vitro Fertilization (IVF)

"Ability is what you're capable of doing, motivation determines what you do, attitude determines how well you do it."
- Lou Holtz

SINCE ITS SUCCESSFUL advent in 1978, IVF has become a well-established treatment for many forms of infertility. Over 1% of all babies born in the United States are thanks to IVF treatment. The pioneer of IVF, Sir Robert Edwards, MD, went on to win the 2010 Nobel Prize in Medicine for his efforts.

An IVF cycle typically includes the following steps or procedures:
- Pretreatment with a hormone pill
  - The pill is frequently an oral contraceptive, or can be a progesterone-only pill (Provera®, Aygestin®).
- Medications (injectables) to grow multiple eggs (ovarian stimulation)
  - The progress in development of follicles will be monitored by blood tests and ultrasounds, which are typically performed early in the morning.
  - Average stimulations proceed for ten days.
  - If few or no follicles develop, the cycle may be cancelled.
- Procedure under anesthesia to extract eggs from the ovary or ovaries (egg retrieval procedure)
  - Under the guidance of a vaginal ultrasound probe, a thin attached needle enters each ovary and sucks out the egg from each follicle.
  - Total procedure takes about 10-20 minutes.

- Insemination of eggs with sperm (fertilization)
  - If eggs are retrieved, they will be fertilized with sperm you provide that same day (Day 0), or with frozen sperm collected previously.
- Development (culture) of any resulting fertilized eggs (embryos) for 2-6 days
  - Done in specialized liquid (culture media) and within incubators that tightly control the temperature and air content (carbon dioxide, oxygen, nitrogen).
  - Since some eggs and embryos may be abnormal, it is expected that not all eggs will fertilize and not all embryos will grow at a normal rate.
- Placement (embryo transfer) of one or more embryo(s) into the uterus
  - Under abdominal ultrasound guidance, a thin tube (catheter) is used to place the embryo(s) in the uterine cavity (no anesthesia is necessary).
  - ASRM has published national guidelines recommending limits on the number of embryos to transfer (see tables below; note that these guidelines are subject to change in the future).
  - These limits differ (favorable vs unfavorable) depending on the stage/quality of embryo development along with the patient's personal history.

Recommended limits on number of 2-3 day old embryos to transfer

Embryos	Age<35	Age 35-37	Age 38-40	Age>40
Favorable	1 or 2	2	3	5
Unfavorable	2	3	4	5

Recommended limits on number of 5-6 day old embryos to transfer

Embryos	Age<35	Age 35-37	Age 38-40	Age>40
Favorable	1	2	2	3
Unfavorable	2	2	3	3

- Support of the uterine lining with hormones (estrogen / progesterone) to permit and sustain pregnancy.
  - ○ Begins after egg retrieval and if a pregnancy results, it is often continued till 9-11 weeks of pregnancy.

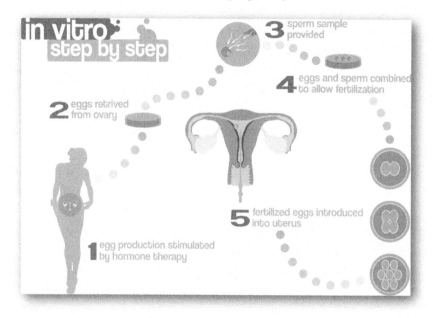

In certain cases, these additional laboratory procedures can be employed:

- Intracytoplasmic sperm injection (ICSI) to increase the chance for fertilization
  - ○ Developed in 1992, this technique involves the isolation of a single sperm followed by microsurgical injection of that sperm into an egg under high-power microscopy.
- Assisted zona hatching (AZH) of embryos to increase the chance of embryo attachment (implantation)
  - ○ Under high-power microscopy, a small opening is made (often via a laser) in the outer shell of the embryo (zona pellucida) to increase the possibility that the embryo will hatch out of its shell and implant in the uterine wall.

- Cryopreservation (freezing) of extra embryos
  ○ Typically, only high quality embryos are frozen.
  ○ Frozen embryos can remain in storage indefinitely without any degradation in quality.
- Cryopreservation (freezing) of eggs
  ○ Newer technology using a technique called vitrification (rapid cooling)
  ○ See Chapter on 'Fertility Preservation'
  ○ Reasons to consider its use:
    ▪ Preserve fertility in women recently diagnosed with cancer who need chemotherapy or pelvic radiation therapy.
    ▪ Impending surgery or ovarian disease associated with risk of damage to ovaries.
    ▪ Risk of premature ovarian insufficiency (e.g., Turner Syndrome, Fragile X Syndrome, family history of premature ovarian insufficiency).
    ▪ Failure to obtain sperm on day of egg retrieval.
    ▪ Preservation of donor eggs.
    ▪ Preservation of fertility to delay pregnancy for personal reasons.

Tips

1. If your tubes are blocked and filled with fluid (hydrosalpinx), it is beneficial to have those tubes surgically removed or disconnected from the uterus. The fluid within the tubes can leak into the uterus and prevent a pregnancy.
2. Being overweight or obese can lower your chance of success from IVF.
3. Current studies indicate that vaginal and intramuscular progesterone have similar efficacy, but oral progesterone is less effective.
4. Vaginal progesterone is absorbed locally and does not impact blood progesterone levels. Avoid looking at progesterone levels if you are using vaginal progesterone.

5. If you have moral or religious objections to discarding embryos, many programs can limit the number of eggs to fertilize and freeze the extra eggs for future use.

Quotes

"Trying to conceive can get really tedious when timing intercourse. I almost enjoyed our IVF cycle because we were told not to have sex (which of course we did because we were told not to) and my hubby only had to give a sample so it took the trying out as far as intercourse and after three years of trying that was really nice."

• • •

"As I sit here I am counting down the days before my IVF procedure I am excited but I am also kind of sad, scared and nervous. I try to think positive but I also prepare myself for the worst."

• • •

"We just completed our first round of IVF and are in the two week wait... the pressure!"

• • •

"On our fourth round of IVF, I got the greatest call on Thanksgiving. Beta was over 100 and finally got a positive from the home pregnancy test. I should be beyond excited and happy. I am so happy but have a constant thought and fear of miscarriage or something going wrong. I'm scared I am going to harm it with all the stress I put on this."

•••

"I am about to try my first round of IVF and feel apprehensive. What if it doesn't work and we spend all this money and emotional investment? I already feel like a failure that all these injectable cycles haven't worked."

•••

"I was super nervous and anxious before my IVF cycle. It got easier as the cycle went through and it goes by pretty quick. The hardest parts for me were just before I started and while waiting for my beta. During the two week wait, keep yourself busy and try not to let yourself dwell on it maybe not having worked. Stay positive and keep up your hope however you have to! It worked for us the first try."

•••

"I had cancer treatment at a young age (21) and had my eggs frozen so I could keep the hope alive of having kids in the future, I am now 29 and my partner and I have decided to start trying next year."

•••

"Not gonna lie, I am pretty excited to have to take it easy for a few days after ER. I have a whole stack of Disney movies and a new cozy blanket waiting for me!"

•••

"I had my WTF meeting with RE this morning to discuss the failed IVF. It went well. He explained he wants to change the protocol for my next cycle because he thinks this may result in better quality, rather than quantity."

•••

"Don't focus so much on embryo grades. My clinic uses a different system than everyone else. My RE told me not to focus on the number because in the grand scheme of things any embryo rating can turn into a pregnancy."

CHAPTER 19

Preimplantation Genetic Screening (PGS)

*"The individual who says it is not possible should move out of
the way of those doing it."*
- Tricia Cunningham

PREIMPLANTATION GENETIC SCREENING (PGS), also sometimes called 'pre-implantation genetic diagnosis (PGD)', is a specialized genetic test used in conjunction with an IVF cycle.

PGS involves a biopsy, or removal, of cells from embryos, followed by preparation of the cells, and subsequent analysis by advanced laboratory techniques. As a result of such analysis, cells with a particular genetic or chromosomal abnormality may be identified. It is assumed that these cells represent the genetic and/or chromosomal make-up of the embryos from which they had been removed. Based upon the results of the genetic analysis, embryos with a suspected abnormality may be excluded from those transferred to the woman's uterus.

To test the cells, an embryologist makes an opening in the covering of the embryo, and removes one or multiple cells from the embryo. The embryo biopsy can be performed at either at the 1-cell stage (polar body biopsy), day 3 of embryo development (blastomere biopsy) or day 5/6 of development (trophectoderm biopsy). It is common for labs to freeze the biopsied embryos, since it can take some time to perform the genetic testing. Once results are obtained, the embryos that tested 'normal' can be transferred in a subsequent cycle.

PGS may be recommended in the following circumstances:

1. Advanced maternal age
2. Known single-gene defect in prospective parents (e.g. Cystic fibrosis, sickle cell)
3. Known chromosomal abnormality in prospective parents (e.g. translocations)
4. Failed Implantation or multiple unsuccessful cycles of IVF
5. Recurrent Miscarriage

Based upon expanding experience with PGS, recommendations for its use are frequently being revised.

Tips

1. Inquire about cost since PGS is usually not covered by insurance, even if IVF is covered.
2. Present evidence indicates that embryo biopsy on day 5 or 6 (blasto-cyst-stage) is superior to day 3 (cleavage-stage) biopsy.
3. Biopsy of embryos under skilled hands (by trained embryologists) does not harm the health of the embryos.

Quotes

"I worry if we do not do the testing that we could end up wasting money and additional emotional stress from negative pregnancy tests on embryos that only appear to be great. "

●●●

"I banked embryos and did PGS testing for each cycle; but I went back and forth about whether it was worth the cost since we did not produce a lot of blastocysts due to my DOR/poor egg quality. Ultimately, I'm glad I chose that option because: 1) I wanted more information on why I couldn't conceive, and it confirmed that poor egg quality was likely the cause; 2) we wanted to do a SET; and 3) I hoped to spare myself the emotional trauma of multiple failed transfers."

• • •

"Some less expensive options for PGS: 1) do multiple rounds, freeze after fertilization, and when you have a sufficient number, let all grow to blast at once, biopsy each and send off the biopsies for testing; or 2) do multiple rounds, grow out each embryo to blast every cycle, freeze the biopsies, and send off the biopsies for testing at one time when you have a sufficient number. (I chose to test after each cycle because I was impatient, and wanted to know how many cycles I needed to do.)"

• • •

"I have to say I took the miscarriage really bad. Looking back, I was kind of going mentally scary crazy. I wouldn't want to go through something like that again. With the PGS testing, I think I have better chances."

• • •

"Did you know that many PGS / PGD labs charge the same fee whether they test 2, 5, or even 8 embryos? Given this, most of them will allow you to "batch" embryos until you have a critical mass to test at once (there's usually a small additional fee to store the biopsy samples in the meantime). So in our case, we're not going to have them run the test this time around, unless we have 4 or more Day 5/6 blasts."

• • •

"I'm glad I did PGS because it has given me some peace of mind about moving on to donor egg. If I hadn't done it, I'd have probably gone through a 2-week wait each time only to be disappointed, or perhaps to have a chemical pregnancy. I'd probably be trying again, too, without this information letting me know why it hasn't worked."

• • •

"A friend of mine had 30 eggs retrieved and had 3 left on Day 5 to biopsy for PGD. Two embryos turned out to be normal and one was abnormal so she implanted one and has a beautiful baby girl now and one is frozen for the future. It only takes one!!"

CHAPTER 20

Fertility Preservation

*"Never say never because limits, like fears, are often just an
illusion."*
- Michael Jordan

WOMEN ARE BORN with a limited number of eggs in their ovaries that con-
tinually decrease throughout their reproductive life. The maximum number
of eggs is about 6-7 million at 20 weeks of gestation as a female fetus. This
number decreases to about 1-2 million at birth; 300,000-500,000 at puberty;
25,000 at age 37 years; and about 1,000 at age 51 years (average age of menopause). Although women continue to ovulate until menopause, the probabil-
ity of achieving a pregnancy decreases as they age because of the fewer and
poorer quality eggs that remain. Besides age, other factors can also increase
the rate of egg loss (e.g., smoking, genetic factors, ovarian surgery, chemotherapy, pelvic radiation).

In order to preserve fertility, the freezing of eggs (oocyte cryopreservation) has recently become a viable option. Even though the first human
birth using a previously frozen egg occurred in 1986, technical challenges
prevented widespread use. More recently however, technology advances in
egg freezing using a process called vitrification (ultra-rapid egg cooling)
has made the process reliable. Once eggs have been vitrified, they can
be stored indefinitely in liquid nitrogen for many years. The process to
obtain the eggs requires a woman to undergo IVF treatment (see Chapter
on IVF).

The following are possible reasons to consider egg freezing:

- Preserve fertility in women recently diagnosed with cancer who need chemotherapy or pelvic radiation therapy.
- Impending surgery or ovarian disease associated with risk of damage to ovaries.
- Risk of premature ovarian insufficiency (e.g., Turner Syndrome, Fragile X Syndrome, family history of premature ovarian insufficiency).
- Failure to obtain sperm on day of egg retrieval.
- Preservation of donor eggs.
- Preservation of fertility to delay pregnancy for personal reasons.

It is estimated that for women ages 30 to 36 years, they may need 12 eggs in storage to ultimately get a live birth, whereas women ages 36-39 may need 30 eggs. Thus, the most appropriate age for effective egg freezing may be in the early-to-mid-30s, before fertility begins to significantly decline.

Tips

1. See an RE if you are in your early 30s and not planning to start a family … you may want to freeze your eggs to preserve your fertility.
2. If you were recently diagnosed with cancer (or know someone) and need chemotherapy or radiation, ask your cancer doctor about preserving your fertility.
3. Several companies are now offering insurance coverage for fertility preservation.

CHAPTER 21

Acupuncture

"Unless you try to do something beyond what you have already mastered, you will never grow."
- Ronald E. Osborn

ACUPUNCTURE IS AN ancient Chinese treatment that involves stimulation of specific acupuncture points along the skin using very thin, single-use, stainless steel needles. It can also be associated with the application of pressure, heat, or laser light to these same points. The needles are inserted painlessly, and used to stimulate certain 'energy points' thought to regulate physical, mental, emotional, and spiritual balance. These energy points are called *Qi* (pronounced "Chee"), that ancient Chinese wisdom says must flow through the body unhampered from head to toe.

There are several small studies on the impact of acupuncture on IVF treatment, with some showing an improvement in pregnancy rates, while others showing no difference. Many fertility centers refer patients for adjunctive therapy with acupuncture, especially for women who have failed one or more attempts with IVF.

Tips

1. Some insurance companies may cover the cost of acupuncture
2. Some acupuncturists have special expertise and experience in dealing with fertility patients
3. High yield times to do acupuncture are close to the time of your embryo transfer procedure (before and after).

Acupuncture

Quotes

"I decided to give acupuncture a try. I figured it can't hurt and I'm becoming a human pincushion anyway."

• • •

"Make sure your acupuncturist is licensed and specializes in infertility. That he/she uses new clean needles (mine were individually wrapped) each time. You can even ask your RE for referral to one."

• • •

"I promise it does NOT hurt! They are super tiny needles. If nothing else, acupuncture is very relaxing."

• • •

"Sometimes insurance will cover, so look into that. Mine was coded as for migraines (which was not a lie. I did go for those too!) so insurance covered all but co-pay."

• • •

"So, I never really did acupuncture until this cycle that I finally got my positive pregnancy test. I did it before and after transfer. I also did it before my second beta. Now, it could totally have been a coincidence that this cycle worked but I can't help but wonder."

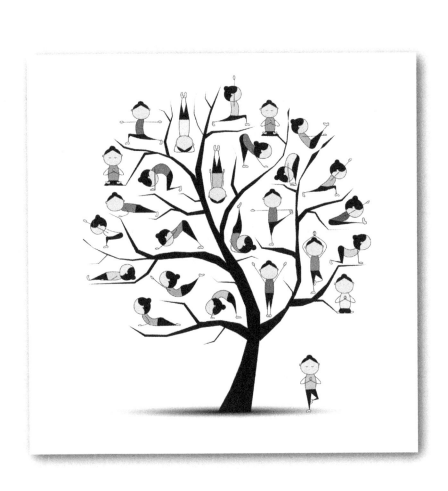

CHAPTER 22

Yoga

"The quieter you become, the more you can hear."
- Ram Dass

YOGA IS AN ancient, spiritual discipline of Indian (Hindu) origin. The word "yoga" comes from the Sanskrit root "yuj", which means "to unite" the spirit and physical body together. Its practice includes breath control (*pranayama*), meditation (*dhyaan*), and the use of specific bodily postures (*asanas*), to harmonize the body with the mind, and thus improve health and relaxation.

There are many different methods of yoga, and hundreds of different yoga poses. Each pose helps to strengthen your mind and body, as well as regain balance between all your bodily functions, including your reproductive system. Yoga can help bring balance to your endocrine system, improve circulation, support your immune system, and bring peace to your conception journey.

Yoga practices aim to engage the movement of *prana* – the innate energy or life force within us. With regard to reproduction, the key is to have free flowing 'apana', which is downward flowing *prana* (energy) centered in the pelvis. Therefore, look for poses to increase *apana*, such as the 'Bridge Pose', 'Mountain Pose', 'Standing Forward Bend', 'Butterfly Pose', 'Childs Pose', and 'Legs Up The Wall Pose'. In addition, certain poses can also relax, soften, and open the pelvis, such as the 'Yogini Squat', 'Bound Angle Pose', 'Seated Twist', 'Goddess Pose' and the 'Corpse Pose'.

The Treatments

Tips

1. Yoga can be started by anyone, even if you don't feel very flexible or strong.
2. Yoga is especially good if your mind is very busy such that you have trouble slowing down to relax. Yoga can help release muscle tension that leads to calming the mind.
3. There are many different types of yoga depending on the teacher. Pick an experienced instructor and a small class (less than 15 people).
4. Hatha yoga is considered good for fertility as it involves slower and flowing movements.
5. Typically, a yoga class at a gym is more focused on the physical benefits, while a class at a yoga center will delve more into the mental and spiritual side.
6. While holding a specific pose, visualize in your mind that a powerful energy is flowing into your pelvis.
7. Remember to practice the breathing exercises in yoga (such as Rhythmic Rapid Breathing, Alternate Nostril Breathing, and Bee Breath), which help calm your mind, purify your body, and allow for smooth flow of *prana*.
8. If your partner is up for it, try doing yoga together as a couple … it can help reconnect the two of you.

Quotes

"I took a yoga class last night. Holy crap I'm out of shape! My arms and hips are so sore this morning."

•••

"Yoga class can be a great way to reduce stress while reminding you of what you looked like before all of this."

• • •

"Yoga is a natural way of calming the mind, focusing on the basics like breathing and decreasing anxiety while increasing flexibility and strength. It helps ground me, which in turn helps with everything."

• • •

"I started doing yoga earlier this year and don't plan on stopping."

• • •

"I am grateful for yoga and all it is teaching me, and for the ways it is preparing my body for pregnancy."

• • •

"You can actually search YouTube and find tons of short workout videos on yoga or pilates. It's awesome because you can find ones that are fit to the time you have. That and its free."

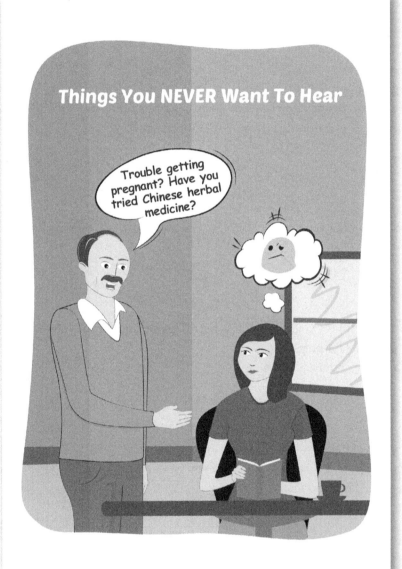

CHAPTER 23

Herbs / Supplements

"It takes nothing to join the crowd. It takes everything to stand alone."
- Hans F. Hansen

THERE IS NO shortage of "natural" over-the-counter herbs and supplements that claim to boost fertility for both women and men. Fertility herbs are made from leaves, bark, roots, flowers, and fruits, and can come in tablet, granule, or tea form.

Although there may be some small promising studies, there is not enough high-quality, published research to show that herbs or supplements are truly beneficial. Furthermore, it is possible that some herbs/supplements may have a harmful effect on the body or the fetus, and some may have a negative interaction with existing fertility medications.

Some common herbs/supplements associated with fertility include chasteberry, red clover, stinging nettle, red raspberry leaves, dong quai root, vitex, black cohosh, false unicorn root, L-arginine, maca root, ashwagandha root, castor oil, Echinacea, and green tea extract. These and others claim to improve various issues ranging from hormonal imbalance, ovulation, endometriosis, miscarriage, reproductive tissue blood flow, and egg/sperm quality.

Tips

1. The Food and Drug Administration (FDA) does not regulate herbs.
2. Chasteberry and Vitex are contraindicated during pregnancy and lactation.

3. Some herbs and supplements may contain hormones that counteract with existing treatment.
4. If you want to try an herbal supplement, check with your fertility doctor.
5. Adequate vitamin D in your system has been correlated with improved odds of pregnancy. Among women of reproductive age, more than 40% are deficient in vitamin D. Have your PCP check your vitamin D level.
6. Avoid using DHEA supplements. At present time, the studies are limited and it may adversely impact your progesterone level.

Quotes

"Nothing out there simply "improves fertility"; everything addresses a particular problem, and if that's not your problem, it'll do nothing at best. It's always advisable to ask your doctor before you take anything; even "natural" stuff and over-the-counter medicine can have side effects and interactions that could be harmful or negatively impact your fertility."

Part Four

The Relationships

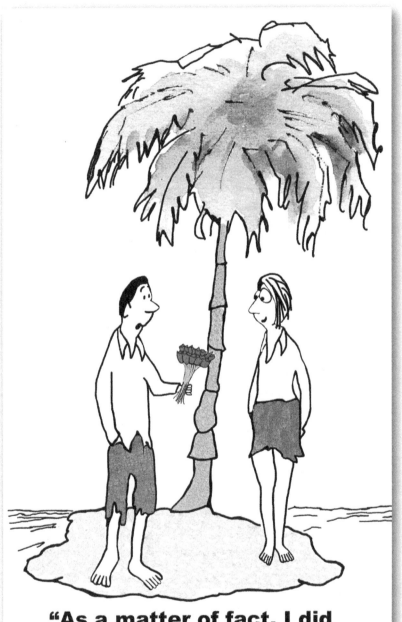

"As a matter of fact, I did get you a Valentine's Day gift."

CHAPTER 24

Partner / Spouse

"You were created to make somebody else's life better. Somebody needs your smile. They need your love, your encouragement and your gifts."
- Unknown

FOR THOSE OF you fortunate to have a partner or spouse, congratulations! Remember, you have already overcome an important life milestone in finding that 'special someone' who is ready to build a family with you.

Many couples go on to assume that when the time is right, they will begin to 'try' and will surely be pregnant based on their calendar. Unfortunately, things don't always go as planned, leading to the taxing and emotionally charged issues associated with infertility. Who else but to frequently take out the stress and frustrations upon … your partner, of course!

Depending on the cause(s) of infertility, guilt and blame start creeping into the relationship. Keep in mind that men and women are different, and handle things differently. Men may take a diagnosis of male factor as a direct hit on their 'manhood' and self-esteem. He may not feel like a 'real man' or embarrassed for 'shooting blanks'. Women may feel guilty and inadequate for not being able to 'give her partner a child'.

Women are more able to talk things out and share feelings with other women, as well as seek out support groups. Men like to solve things and are more apt to try and work things out on their own. Women may seek out a lot more information from extraneous sources such as websites, books, blogs, and chat rooms. Men may more likely rely on information received primarily from the doctor's visit. Women may find themselves saying things like "Why am I the only one doing any research" or "Clearly having a baby is more important to me" or "I have to do all the work". Men may say things like "It's not my fault" or "Just relax".

Remember, you are a TEAM. BOTH of you care for each other and want the exact same thing. BOTH of you are stressed and frustrated. BOTH of you need to understand and support each other.

Tips

1. Infertility is not a 'fault' of anyone … it is a medical condition.
2. Male-factor infertility is just as common as female-factor infertility.
3. Blame never works.
4. Take time to go out on regular 'dates' to re-connect with your spouse.
5. Men generally want to help/support their partners --- they are not mind-readers, so let them regularly know what you need.
6. Seek help and counseling early.
7. Support groups can be a good source of comfort and reassurance that you are not alone.

Quotes

"Sex went from intimacy to I don't want to look at you again. It's hard to be open with it all but there is more support and understanding than people initially think. Take your time and use your husband for support and know communication is huge between you guys."

• • •

"When my husband and I first met in college, we were all over each other and trying to prevent pregnancy ... and now we're like, ugh, time to do it again!"

•••

"It is very common for the guys to be über-practical and zero emotional when we're at our most emotional. It's how they deal with things. It can be maddening at times but it can be really helpful if you choose to look at it that way."

•••

"Men don't understand. Same way women who have never had fertility issues don't understand. I would research and read everything I could to him, but he still has no clue how most things work in the fertility world. He felt like it was his job to "fix" things and all I wanted was his support, a shoulder to cry on, and a hand to hold."

•••

"My wife and i have 7 and 1/2 years of marriage under our belt and 6 miscarriages. It's been hell trying to deal with all the emotions. She has told me many time that I should leave her and find a woman that can give me the children I deserve and I keep telling her that I married her when she had no kids and I'll die with her if she has no kids. I also tell her that if it never happens, then we get to retire a lot earlier!!"

•••

"My husband didn't even want to do IUI or IVF at first. But he knew how much we both wanted a baby, so it was worth the work and the cost. And let's face it, the woman is the one who has to go through the most, physically. Like giving yourself shots daily!"

•••

"I have been married to my husband for one year. He is very supportive... especially with Clomid® mood swings... I just remind him that it is God's way of preparing him for the pregnancy mood swings."

•••

"My husband and I are trusting God to give us a miracle now, either naturally or through adoption. The one bit of advice I would like to share, is you and your husband are a team, you will rely and need each other through this process and despite the outcome, you will weather it better as a team."

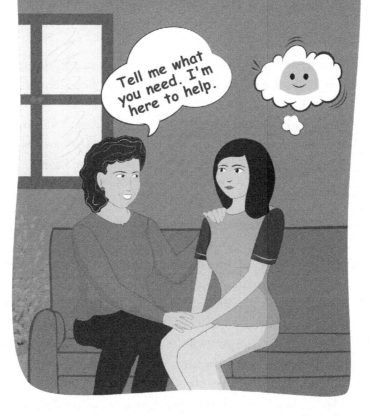

CHAPTER 25

Family

"In family life, love is the oil that eases friction, the cement that binds closer together, and the music that brings harmony."
- Eva Burrows

FAMILY SURROUNDS so many of us. Even if they are not in the same town, with the use of technology and social media, it may often seem as if they are living with us at times.

As much as family members can be a source of strength, inspiration, and guidance, most everyone has families that are not "perfect" and can increase the stress and pressure of having a child. When it comes to having children, it is common to hear things like, 'When are you going to start trying" or "Don't wait too long" or "Why don't you have kids yet". Furthermore, you may have siblings who are already pregnant or have several children ... all as if they got pregnant with ease.

Infertility is certainly a personal and sensitive issue. Remember that you don't owe anyone an explanation and share only as much as you feel comfortable. It is very reasonable to politely answer inquiring minds with "Working on it" or "We will keep you posted". Alternatively, you can let family know that it is a stressful topic, and you will let them know when you are ready to discuss again. Being honest about your feelings may help them understand.

Keep in mind that others may also think they are being helpful by offering advice. They are not trying to be insensitive or say hurtful things, even though it may come across that way. Consider confiding with select members who you feel close to and know they have your best interest at heart. Stay positive and know that your family loves you.

Family

Quotes

"Happy Mother's Day -- it comes around every year; but when you have empty arms, it's very hard to hear. It's a day to celebrate a mother, for all the trials she has overcome; but a reminder to me of my loneliness and shame."

• • •

"Even if family are supportive about treatment, they will nag you about every little progress you and your wife make throughout the process. If you're not getting good news from your doctor, you don't really want to talk about it with anybody except with your spouse. My husband and I kept it to ourselves and it's the best decision we ever made."

• • •

"Unfortunately, people are so cruel and don't realize how much they can hurt us with their "baby talk or making advice"."

• • •

"I don't have anyone in my family or close friends that have any idea what I'm going through with infertility. They just don't understand what this is like."

• • •

"Holidays are sheer torture for infertile couples. Having endured years of them and watching every married sibling and cousin procreate (and announce in cutesy ways at Christmas), I can tell you it is painful. Last Christmas, our family spent a week at the beach together. While others had gone out to the beach/pool, I stayed in the condo with my 20-month old niece who had fallen asleep in my arms. While she slept, I cried. I realized how badly I wanted my own to do this with."

• • •

"I feel like everyone and their mom has been asking me 'when are you guys trying for #2'? I always say something like 'we are really enjoying our little guy right now' and then they all say 'well don't wait too long!' If I tell them about our journey with infertility (we have been on injectable since last May), they say things like 'women always get pregnant easily the second time around.' Um, I CAN'T OVULATE. I will NEVER get pregnant on my own. People just don't understand."

• • •

"We didn't tell my family right away because we weren't sure of what their response would be. They tend to joke and poke fun at things … I think it's because they don't understand. But when he did tell my mom and dad, they were very supportive. They encouraged us to try if that was what we wanted. Both our parents are not sad that we can't give them grand-children … they are sad that their own children have to go through this sadness."

• • •

"It's so frustrating. EVERYONE around me is popping out kids and getting pregnant. It's so unfair! We struggle so much for a slim possibility. And the questions …. I don't want to share my business with everyone but they just keep asking. So you guys having kids? Why aren't you pregnant yet? You would think that 5 years and they would stop asking. Nope. *Sigh*."

• • •

"I've been accused of jealousy and wanting others pregnancies to fail since I haven't had one with my husband yet. The fact that it's family makes it so much worse. And of course food and sodas get pushed onto me and they don't get why I can't. It's frustrating."

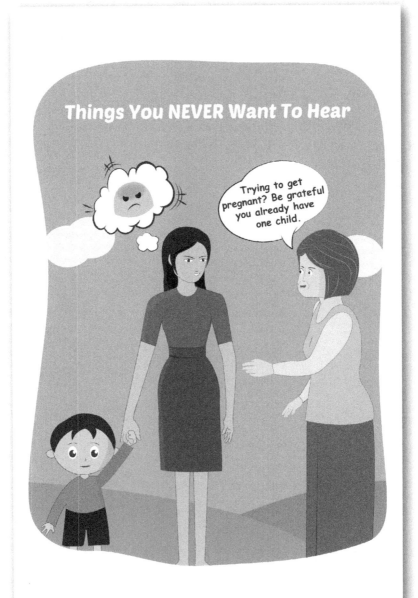

CHAPTER 26

Religion

"Be kind, be fair, be honest, be true, and all of these things will come back to you."
- Unknown

RELIGION PLAYS AN integral part in the lives of so many individuals. It can be a source of identity, comfort, and spiritual guidance. Even within a particular religion, many interpretations and practice patterns exist. For many couples dealing with infertility, their religion provides them an important sense of hope and faith that they will soon be blessed with a child.

Many religions also have much to say about how to manage fertility and reproduction. It can therefore lead to various positive and negative feelings about infertility and its treatment options.

Do be open with your fertility doctor about your religious beliefs and feelings during your initial consult. It is very likely that you are not the first one to present with such beliefs. Many of your fears can be alleviated after discussing options that will meet your needs and belief systems.

Tips

1. If your religious belief does not allow for the discarding of excess embryos, talk to your fertility doctor. They can limit the number of eggs to fertilize, and extra eggs can be frozen.
2. If you already have extra embryos frozen and no longer need them, consider donating them to another couple.

3. Don't be afraid to ask your doctor to pray with you (regardless of his/her religious beliefs).
4. Infertility impacts couples of all religious beliefs. Talk to other trusted family and friends about how to balance your beliefs with fertility treatment.
5. This is YOUR life --- live it the way it makes sense to YOU.
6. Miracles happen every single day!

Quotes

"The worst part about all this though is my Dad, who is super Catholic, is against IVF and started talking about how it would put a wedge between us. Don't get me wrong, I am not letting that discourage me from getting it, but it would be nice to have support from my own father during what is easily the most difficult time in my life."

• • •

"My husband is Catholic and talked to his very conservative priest when we were about to do IVF. The priest encouraged us to do IVF, and said that the Church wasn't opposed to medical assistance in starting life, but in ending it. So really the fear was about what would happen to unused embryos."

• • •

"Just my opinion, if you are religious, the IVF process is still VERY much in the hands of God. IVF is no guarantee of conception or a successful pregnancy. God is present in the process; in fact, I think we see him even more clearly in it!"

• • •

"I try to have as much faith in myself to stat strong and pray that someday I will get pregnant."

• • •

"I feel like I am a much more bitter person that I ever was. I hate going ANYWHERE because I will always see a pregnant woman (or 5) and become upset. My husband and I were watching a comedian on TV who was talking about how blessed he and his wife were for having two wonderful children and I lost it. I am a Christian, but this is very trying!!!!!! When will I get to have this blessing? Will I ever? Am I less blessed without children?"

• • •

"I know, although, I don't have a baby yet, this process has made me a whole lot more sensitive, understanding that I am not in control, God is, and that it's up to me how I let others affect me."

• • •

"Sometimes you can't help but say "Why me God?" I know I have, I begged to get pregnant for my birthday then this Christmas. Heck, I can't even get my body to ovulate!!"

• • •

"We pray to God with all our heart and in the end any child we have, biological or adopted, belongs to the Lord anyway and will only be on loan to us until we visit him in heaven ourselves."

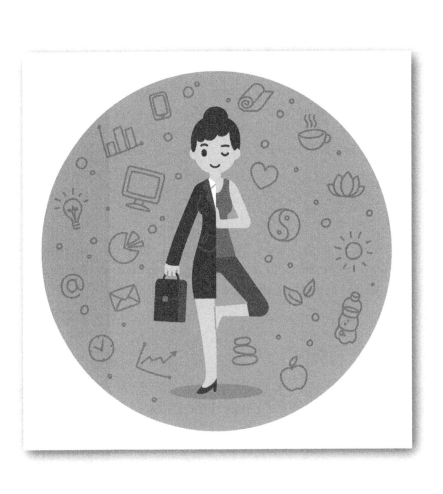

CHAPTER 27

Job / Career

"It always seems impossible until it is done."
- Nelson Mandela

THERE ARE MORE women in the workplace today than ever before. Career and work are important in many ways and are often a source of self-identity and self-esteem. Many women fear telling their boss or co-workers about their fertility struggles due to fears of discrimination or not getting promoted. Fertility treatment may also need adjustments in work schedules.

Remember there are laws against discrimination in the workplace. Ironically, many women find support and comfort in the workplace by sharing their struggles with trusted colleagues. It is not uncommon for other co-workers to be going thru similar issues. Finding such support can certainly ease the added pressure and stress of balancing work and fertility treatment.

Tips

1. Most fertility centers do early morning monitoring (ultrasound and bloodwork) to accommodate women with job obligations
2. Consider fertility preservation at a younger age (via egg freezing) if you want to delay child-bearing due to career aspirations
3. Talk to your Human Resources (HR) department to find out about options in adjusting your work hours as well as health insurance coverage for fertility treatment

Quotes

"I had one coworker explain that she and her husband decided to take a break so she relaxed and did a bunch of horse riding and that was what did it! I suppose I could've gone into a cost analysis of owning a horse vs. IVF, but I was too exhausted at that point."

• • •

"I am so stressed out at work and worried I may lose my job. I need to take off random times for my IVF treatments and I don't feel great. It's hard for me to travel for work and I have to keep making excuses. I used to love my job but now I am struggling trying to balance it all."

• • •

"I'm currently 14 weeks pregnant, via IVF/PGD and working. I didn't tell my boss yet, as I wanted to wait the end of the first trimester. My performance at work is outstanding (see pregnancy doesn't cause brain freeze!) and I want to ask for a raise based of my increasing responsibilities and better results. I don't intend to be sneaky or unfair, as I want to keep my job, and still have a nice relationship with my boss, but I don't know which one comes first? Also my due date is around the time, my company performs performance reviews. I just want a fair treatment, and not being penalized because pregnant, or take advance of my situation. Would I ask for a raise first, and then after the holidays I will tell him, I'm pregnant?"

• • •

"I told my boss right away about my successful pregnancy, partly because I was afraid that if I had a miscarriage I'd be a mess and need a little of time off to deal with things. That said, no business can discriminate against you just because you're pregnant."

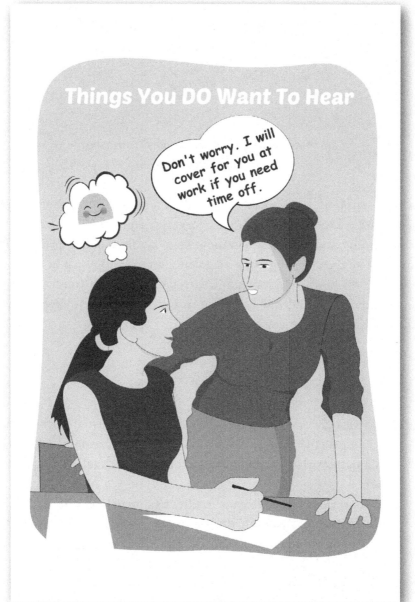

CHAPTER 28

Friends

"Friends are the family we choose for ourselves."
- Edna Buchanan

UNLIKE FAMILY, WE can choose our friends. They are also frequently around us and can be a source of support. As goes with family however, friends can also seem nosy and ask questions about your family building plans. It may also seem like they are all getting pregnant with ease. Do keep in mind that many may also have undergone similar struggles as you. If you have a friend who you know has undergone fertility treatment, seek their support. They will really KNOW what you are going thru.

Tips

1. There may still be a perceived stigma associated with infertility, especially within certain cultures/ethnic groups. Opening a dialogue with a trusted friend about your struggles can go a long way.
2. If your friend has undergone fertility treatment, you will benefit from their emotional support. Keep in mind, however, that their medical issues and treatment outcomes may not apply to you.

Friends

Quotes

"I have so many friends who are pregnant and every single one of them got pregnant easily and quickly."

• • •

"It's hard for friends to understand. And, not to mention the great comments I get ... like 'just relax and you will get pregnant!'"

• • •

"Friends not knowing the struggle I have been through and how much I have thought about it and prayed every night … just to find out I am INFERTILE and without IVF I will always be motherless is something they will never comprehend."

• • •

"I have had one friend tell me silly things like after sex get a pillow and prop it under my back. I'm SCREAMING on the inside, "IF YOUR TUBES ARE DAMAGED YOU CAN STAND ON YOUR HEAD AND NOTHING WILL HAPPEN." But, I simply smile on the outside and cry on the inside."

• • •

"I have JUST started telling close friends what's going on because I felt so alone and like I was going to reach a breaking point. They finally convinced me to do an IUI this cycle. I'm scared but hope for good results. Let's do this!"

•••

"My friend doesn't know the difference between IUI and IVF, even though I've explained it several times! It's hard because I know she's only trying to be supportive, but sometimes I think I need to omit any details and just talk to her on her level. "Yes, we're trying. Having sex with the socks on and standing on my head afterward. I'll let you know when it works.""

•••

"There are so many people who mean well, but that just don't truly understand and so say things that don't really even make sense to those of us that truly get it. Don't let them discourage you from your goal."

•••

"Yesterday my neighbor and good friend asked me if I have thought about seeing a therapist to help me move on after my miscarriage. It has been 4 weeks and she expects me to be all sunshine and rainbows. Just because she got pregnant at the drop of a hat doesn't mean that she is the eternal expert at grieving."

•••

"My close friends have really been great. They try their best to sympathize with me...even though they don't understand. The friend who emailed me regarding her new pregnancy news was really sweet about it also. It is harder to deal with when it is someone close to you, like my friend where I work. I have to see her every day and watch her go through the excitement of her pregnancy. That is what is hard. I find myself having an emotional breakdown at least once a week. I agree that God is in control, it's just hard to explain that to your heart. It's something that I have to deal with one day at a time."

•••

"I feel okay talking to my friends about my infertility, but I know that they can't really understand, although they may sympathize. What really drives me nuts is the one friend I have who accidentally got pregnant at seventeen and now, not even a year after having her first baby, she's pregnant again and feels free to give me advice on how to cope with trying to conceive. I haven't said anything mean or snarky to her in response, but I sure have been tempted!"

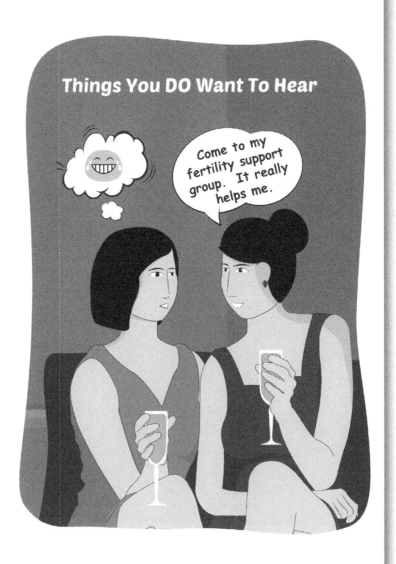

CHAPTER 29

Counseling / Support Groups

"Be kind, for everyone you meet is fighting a hard battle."
- Plato

You ARE NOT alone in dealing with infertility, and you should certainly not feel alone. Dealing with infertility brings complex feelings and can impact not only how you feel about yourself, but also your relationships with your partner, family, and friends. The benefits of support from others while going thru fertility treatment can be significant, and help improve your chances of success.

Support from a mental health professional (fertility counselor, social worker, psychologist, psychiatrist, marriage therapist) should be especially considered if you are feeling anxious, depressed, or finding it hard to live your life productively. The following list of signs can serve as a guide to seeking counseling: marital issues, loss of interest in daily activities, difficulty concentrating, social isolation, persistent feelings of guilt or worthlessness, difficulty sleeping, changes in weight, increased alcohol or drug use, thoughts of suicide.

Support can also come from discussions with family members, friends, or work colleagues. Given that infertility is very common, it is quite likely that several people in your family and social circle are dealing with or have experienced similar issues.

There are also several support groups that can help. You can find groups that meet in person close to you or join an on-line support group. Knowing others going through the same issues can make a huge difference. Here are a few to consider:

1. RESOLVE: The National Infertility Association (www.resolve.org)
   A non-profit, charitable organization founded in 1974, who works to improve the lives of women and men living with infertility. RESOLVE provides community to these women and men, connecting them with others who can help, empowering them to find resolution. RESOLVE provides free support programs in communities nationwide, leads efforts to increase public education and reduce the stigma around infertility and promises to protect legal access to all family building options.

2. Fertility Within Reach (www.fertilitywithinreach.org)
   A non-profit organization founded in 2011 that aims to empower infertile individuals to advocate in order to build their family. The organization provides information to support your communication process with physicians, insurance companies, employers, and legislators in your efforts to access Infertility treatment for yourself and the infertility community.

3. Fertile Hope (www.livestrong.org/fertilehope)
   A Livestrong Foundation initiative, dedicated to helping women and men understand risks and options related to cancer treatment and fertility. They provide tools and resources to evaluate your risks and options, and help with accessing discounted rates for fertility preservation and finding local fertility-related resources.

4. Frank Talk (www.franktalk.org)
   A non-profit, on-line community of men who are fighting erectile dysfunction (ED). The site strives to advance patient education about ED and provides a place to talk to other men about their journey.

5. Choice Moms (www.choicemoms.org)
   Provides resources, connections, and support for single women who are choosing to become mothers.

Counseling / Support Groups

Tips

1. Seek emotional help/support early and often. Balancing the mind is an important component of the infertility journey.
2. You will learn more than you expected from talking to others about your infertility experience.

Quotes

"I haven't told any of my friends that we're seeing an infertility specialist and even haven't told my mom, who I'm very close with, about it. I don't know if it's embarrassment or just not wanting to talk about our 'problems'."

• • •

"So I think we were hesitant to tell some people because of the reaction or them wanting to give "tips" that really won't help us. It's really personal, and then to have your aunt telling you how to conceive? It's laughable really. But we didn't hold back because of shame. There's nothing to be ashamed of. It's not your fault. We were just dealt cards and we have to deal with it."

• • •

"I went to a social worker when my husband and I were struggling, and I remember the very first appointment, I walked out of there feeling like the sun was shining brighter."

• • •

"After a miscarriage, I personally found therapy very very helpful! I have told people about it and said how it helped me. But I would never flat out say, "You need therapy!" since you can never know what is going on inside another person's head."

• • •

"My therapist was a total lifesaver and really helped me to find ways to move forward while learning to accept my grief and sadness."

• • •

"We have told several people. I told my mom in hopes that she would stop pressuring me to give her a grandbaby. I have also told my coworkers because I will have to miss work and due to the nature of his job all the guys there know too. I find it helpful that they know at work because it is on my mind so much and I spend so much time with them. I'm able to talk about everything and they are so supportive, especially my boss. She went through infertility many years ago and understands how it feels."

• • •

"Counseling is best, because there is a third party who is objective and can help you articulate your feeling/concerns."

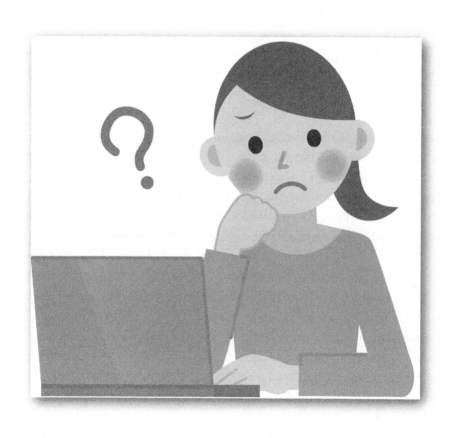

CHAPTER 30

Internet

"If you don't build your dream, someone else will hire you to help them build theirs."
- Tony A. Gaskins, Jr.

THE MAJORITY OF infertility patients go on-line in order to access medical information. Furthermore, many also use the Internet for social support via discussion groups, chat rooms, email, and social media. Depending on the amount and frequency of Internet use, the outcome can range from beneficial to confusing to overwhelming.

I recommend sticking to well-established educational sites to ensure receiving credible information. One of the most comprehensive and reputable sites is www.reproductivefacts.org. It is run by ASRM and provides up-to-date and evidence-based information.

If you read or participate in discussion groups / chat rooms, keep in mind that every patient has their own journey related to their own individual set of issues. Furthermore, there is significant variability within how different fertility specialists practice medicine. The treatment(s) and outcome(s) of one patient may not apply to your situation. If you find that your stress level is increasing after reading online experiences, consider taking a break.

Tips

1. It is common to feel overwhelmed by the process, and to seek help online. Set limits to the time you spend online.
2. Do not make any medical or dietary changes based solely on information you read online. Talk to your RE first.

Internet

Quotes

"Every time I turn around another friend is announcing their pregnancy on Facebook."

•••

"As I read the online forms and posts, and have witnessed others go through it 1, 2 and sometimes even 3 IVF cycles, I think those individuals are very strong. I can't imagine the anticipation each month or cycle, hoping and wishing for a positive test. However, when you want something so bad I guess you must not give up."

•••

"My husband is not for IVF due to the cost, and we have to drive 100 miles for treatment. He doesn't understand how emotional infertility is to me; that's why I use discussion groups because everyone on here gets it."

•••

"I'm so incredibly tired of reading statuses on Facebook from mothers who complain about their children. How "their kids are driving them nuts, etc." Some of us would kill to have a little one running around! If I'm ever fortunate enough to have a child, I vow to never complain about them."

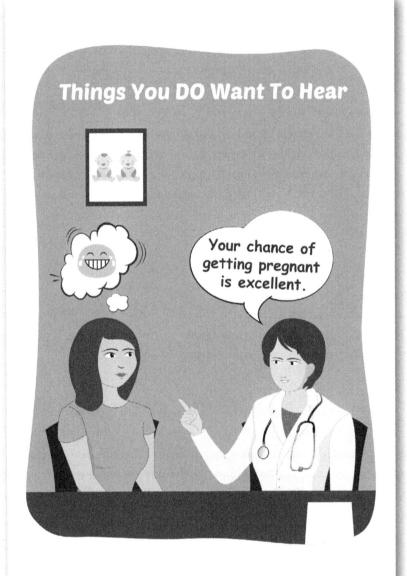

CHAPTER 31

Fertility Nurse

*"To do what nobody else will do, a way that nobody else can do
in spite of all we go through; is to be a nurse."*
- Rawsi Williams

FERTILITY NURSES ARE special individuals and will play a major role during your fertility journey. You will have their phone number on speed-dial. They will be communicating with you frequently, holding your hand, giving you hugs, and guiding you thru the treatment plan laid out by your doctor. A high percentage of the nurses are also trained to perform your ultrasounds and intra-uterine insemination (IUI) procedures.

Many fertility nurses began their career in general obstetrics and have even worked on labor and delivery units in hospitals. Some of the nurses may have also been former infertility patients and know first-hand what you are going thru.

Get to know your nurse well, and know that they are on your side. They will work tirelessly to help you achieve your dream of parenthood.

Tips

1. Fertility nurses have your best interest in mind. They are your biggest advocates.
2. Nurses love to get little gifts such as flowers, cookies, snacks, or thank-you cards. Such acts of gratitude will touch their heart and energize them.

3 Even after you have 'graduated' from the fertility center with a successful pregnancy, do come back to visit your fertility nurse (and doctor). There is no better feeling for them to see you happy, and especially holding your newborn baby!

Quotes

"I have long known why I work in this field. Because, I can think of no higher honor than helping intelligent couples who place their trust in us to help coax forth nothing short of a miracle. Because when I work alongside patients, I get to experience the best and most enchanting moments that life has to offer -- service to those who are desperate to have the privilege to become parents."

• • •

"I've learned over the years that it's okay to simply be with people and especially patients. Despite the overwhelming American preference for extroverts and gabbing, I love silence, which affords healing, contemplation and a deeper understanding of certain situations than can ever be gleaned from gab."

• • •

"Fertility is not an exact science. Answers are not always clear cut. I have had to adjust the way I talk to patients to ensure I do not tell them anything that may contradict what others may have told them."

• • •

"As new developments and scientific advances continue, keeping informed is not only a challenge but also our responsibility as nurses. Networking and attending symposiums provide a unique opportunity for us to learn and share ideas. It is reassuring to talk with other nurses and discover that they too have days in the clinic when they are 'running around like ants on a sticky bun'! In fact, many of us thrive in that kind of environment. Just know that each ant on that sticky bun has a specific goal and a plan for achieving that goal."

• • •

"I continue to work in this field knowing that it is very stressful on my patients. Some women may not feel supported by their partners. Some have not told anyone about their fertility treatment so I am the only one they can call. I am here to support you. I am here to reassure you during the difficult times and here to celebrate when things go well."

• • •

"The support and skill we as nurses bring to our patients and colleagues may very likely change and enhance their lives. What we do matters. We touch the lives of so many people and influence them in so many ways. Empathy, kind words, a positive attitude, respectful interaction, taking the time to listen, maintaining a healthy sense of humor and remembering to smile are contributions we can make every day."

• • •

"One of the most common side effects of IVF medications us nurses hear about from our patients is bloating. Drinking water is one great way to reduce bloat. While it may seem counterintuitive, drinking water actually helps flush your body of excess fluids. Light exercise such as walking can also decrease that uncomfortable feeling. Take comfort in knowing this is a temporary side effect and won't last forever."

• • •

"As an IVF nurse, I provide information, education, and support that enables my patients to make decisions in what most patients see as a very difficult process. By empowering my patients, I allow them to regain some control of their personal situation and feel that they are part of the team."

• • •

"Please don't forget me during holiday time, and send me a picture of that cute baby we helped create! It means more than you know."

Part Five

Every Day

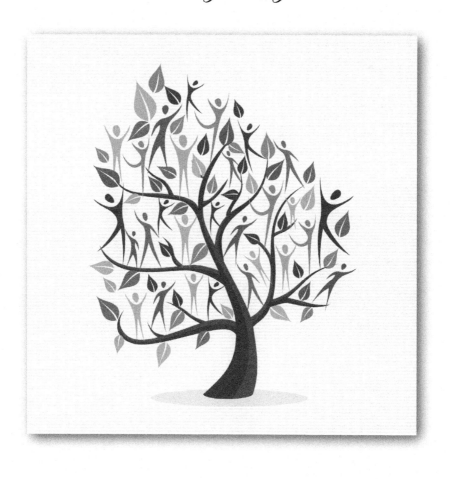

CHAPTER 32

Daily Life

> *"Go confidently in the direction of your dreams. Live the life you have imagined."*
> - Henry David Thoreau

LIVING WITH INFERTILITY can be a daily challenge. The desire to have a child is intense and extraordinary. Normally uneventful things like seeing kids playing outside or eating in a restaurant can become difficult and emotional. Being invited to a friend's baby shower or learning that your friend is pregnant will take all your strength to break a smile and be happy for them.

Nevertheless, seek help early from your doctor and/or nurse. Gain strength from the various support systems described elsewhere in this book. Have faith in the process and know that you will soon be on the other side.

Tips

1. Never think you are alone in dealing with infertility. Communicate often about your struggles with close family and/or friends.
2. Life can be difficult at times, but remember there is always someone who has it worse than you.
3. Keep yourself occupied (work, hobbies, family, social events, etc.) to avoid over-focusing on your fertility issues.
4. Daily exercise will help keep you balanced.
5. Focus on all the good in your life.
6. Take care of yourself – do things you enjoy and that help you relax. Ask others close to you for help when you need a break.

Every Day

Quotes

"I live with the fear and thought that I will never have a child every day."

• • •

"I'd love to go away for a few days to gather myself and relax a bit but I'm scared I'll miss some all-important window!"

• • •

"What I tell myself is that because we had to work so hard to get our little baby here I will appreciate the child more and cherish motherhood much more than others. I don't know if that's the truth or not, but it helps sometimes."

• • •

"I really want to have a baby and I buy baby things now and again. I just can't help myself, although when I look at them I cry!"

• • •

"It's reassuring to be around people who know exactly how this feels. Like I told my husband, I wish someone had a way of telling me that in maybe 1, 2 5, etc. years this will all be a memory and we will have our family. I think the worst thing is the waiting. And it didn't help today to go to a toy store to look for a baby present for my cousin -- all the pregnant bellies in town were there!"

• • •

"I hate going out anymore because it seems everyone can get pregnant except me. I am Catholic and we went to church last night...there was a baptism and I started to cry. My husband keeps tissues on hand these days because he never knows when I will lose it."

CHAPTER 33

Meals And Nutrition

"Take care of your body. It's the only place you have to live."
- Jim Rohn

THERE IS A lot of information and attention placed on our diet, especially when it comes to fertility. Everybody seems to have an opinion on what diets are helpful, especially friends and family members.

To avoid becoming dizzy from all the chatter, here are the key points to remember:

1. Your body weight is critical to optimizing your fertility and pregnancy. Being under- or over-weight has a negative impact on your success. Work towards achieving a BMI between 20-25.
2. Avoid alcohol and caffeine. One alcoholic drink or 1-2 8-ounce cups of coffee per day however, may still be okay while you are trying to get pregnant.
3. Avoid processed foods.
4. Eat bright-colored fruits and vegetables daily (like blueberries, strawberries, red peppers, mango, pineapple, spinach and kale). They are packed with vitamins, minerals, and anti-oxidants.
5. Don't forget your pre-natal vitamin. Keep in mind, however, that this is not a substitute for a balanced and healthy diet.
6. Low-mercury fish can be beneficial due to their high content of omega-3 fatty acids. Women trying to conceive can safely eat up to 12 ounces a week of seafood such as salmon, shrimp, canned light

tuna, or catfish. Avoid high-mercury fish such as grouper, marlin, swordfish, mackerel, shark, and albacore/white tuna.

7. Foods to avoid completely: raw sushi, soft cheese from raw milk, smoked seafood, and refrigerated meat spreads. Also, don't eat food that has been sitting outside for over two hours.

8. Men can also benefit from a multi-vitamin with zinc and selenium – these minerals can help with sperm development.

Tips

1. As your primary care physician (PCP) for a referral to see a nutritionist. They can really help you set up a healthy diet that works for you.

2. Make sure your PCP has checked your Vitamin D level, and provided adequate supplementation if needed. Adequate vitamin D in your system has been correlated with improved odds of pregnancy.

Quotes

"I had been on the Chinese fertility diet while trying to conceive. Only drinking warm teas, no gluten, no dairy and no refined sugar (except the occasional piece of chocolate of course)."

• • •

"Goodness knows I need to lose weight, and if tailoring my diet towards stuff they say helps infertility, I'm game."

• • •

"I plan on starting maca, bee pollen, royal jelly, and CoQ10 beginning next cycle. I also have been drinking dong quai tea for the last month or so."

•••

"I don't have the best embryo quantity response, but I have excellent quality per my RE. I took royal jelly, CoQ10, L-arginine, wheatgrass, fish oil, baby aspirin and selenium."

•••

"I drank wheatgrass for about 3 months but after my last failed IUI in August, I stopped drinking it."

•••

"I am overwhelmed by the information on Google. I'm seriously thinking about trying gluten free or paleo but just don't know where to start."

•••

"I have been trying to step up my healthy eating a bit. I generally eat pretty cleanly, but do eat lunch out a few times a week, occasionally fast food. I am trying to avoid the fast food and I have cut the caffeine/artificial sweeteners (I usually have 1-2 Diet sodas a week)."

•••

"I'm doing fertility diet- basically 90grams of protein and not low carbs but keeping that in check with Mediterranean diet influences (olives, olive oil, artichoke hearts) and also coconut oils and avocado."

•••

"There is no magic fertility diet. Eat a balanced diet and limit crap foods."

•••

"I tend to stick with just water. I've learned my body takes any sugars and converts it to fat quickly. So juices are a no go for me unless I add fiber and that's just not tasty."

•••

"I went gluten free about 4-5 months ago. I have never felt better! My inflammation is down, I was losing weight (recently had an attack on Peppermint Patties), and I have no more headaches."

•••

"I eat mostly protein and veggies. I'm staying away from bread, pasta, dairy, and refined sugars, along with caffeine. Also staying away from fried foods and high fat foods. I've lost 16 pounds in 1 month."

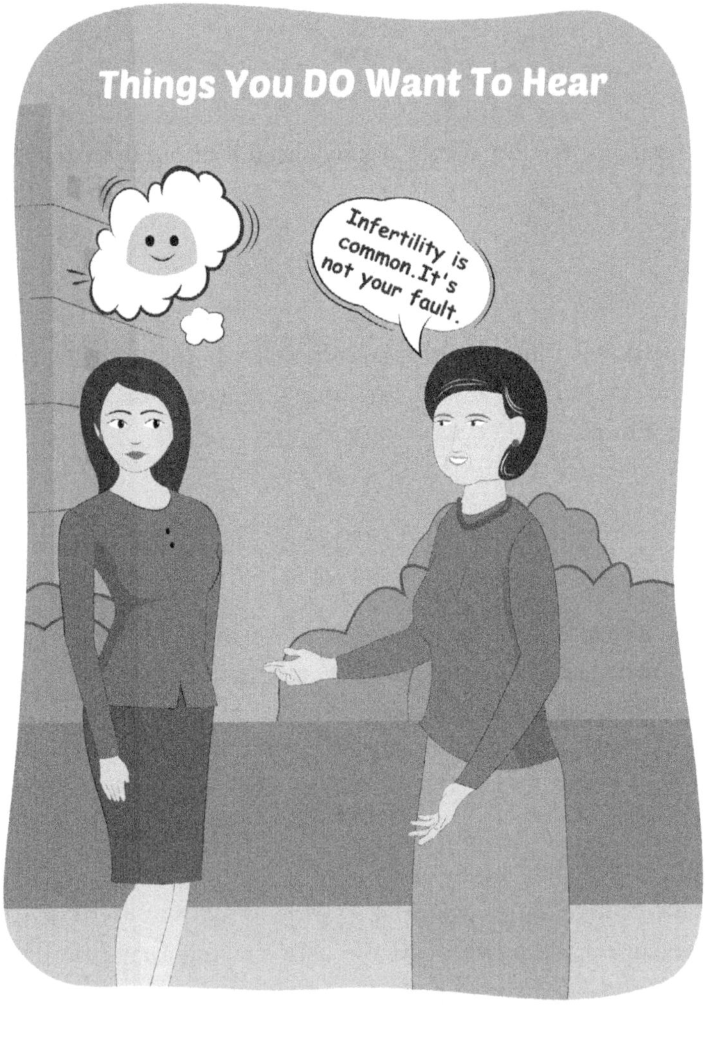
Things You DO Want To Hear
Infertility is common. It's not your fault.

CHAPTER 34

Feeling Different

"The way to control a bull is to give it a big pasture."
- Zen proverb

STRUGGLING TO HAVE a child can lead to many issues, including the feeling of being different ... thoughts like being "not good enough", "inadequate", or "empty" are common. Some cultural belief systems may even increase or intensify such thoughts.

Women often blame themselves for not being able to have a child or feel others may be blaming them for the same. This can lead to isolation, sadness and even depression.

Know that these feelings are common and you are not alone. Communicate your thoughts and feelings, rather than letting them build up inside you. The process of coming to terms with such feelings can be gradual, but begin by knowing who you are, loving yourself, and realizing that with proper medical help ... success can be realized.

Tips

1. Express your feelings via not only communicating with family or friends, but also by keeping a diary of your fertility journey.

2. Your significant other / spouse may be having similar feelings ... talk to and support each other.

3. If you find yourself feeling sad, talk to your physician or nurse about counseling, joining a support group, or joining activities with others that may offer a support structure.

Every Day

Quotes

"Remember to stay in YOUR experience ... Not anyone else! Every person is so different from each other...resist comparing yourself to others ... it's not fair to you or them. Hormones, egg quality, sperm issues, age! So many factors for each person. Don't look in the rear view mirror. Focus on your lane, your fertility vehicle...put in good gas, oil, attitude and don't waste time looking around at the other cars on the road. You can't control them...only your vessel...to some degree."

• • •

"If we conceive, my first inclination is not to tell anyone that we used Clomid®/IUI because I don't want that to be the caveat to the topic of our child/children."

• • •

"I'm feeling terribly bad about myself today. I splurged and had a few (more than 2) glasses of wine last night, then cried because I hated myself for it. I had decided not to drink anything at all this cycle (last cycle I had 1-2 here and there during my stimulations). I'm sure it's not a huge deal but I've decided it's not worth the guilt I feel afterwards, so that was my one free pass."

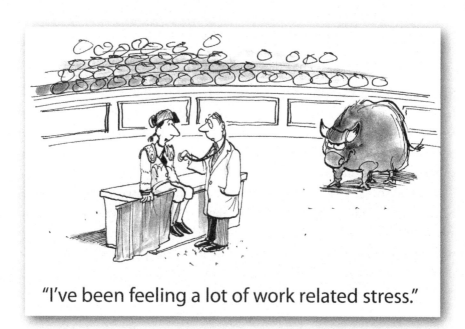

"I've been feeling a lot of work related stress."

CHAPTER 35

Stress

"You don't always need a plan. Sometimes you just need to breathe, trust, let go and see what happens."
- Mandy Hale

STRESS IS UNIVERSAL. Everyone feels stress from time to time at varying levels. It is your body's way of responding to any kind of need, threat, or demand. When you feel threatened, your nervous system responds by releasing numerous stress hormones, such as cortisol and epinephrine (adrenaline), which put your body in action mode.

Not all stress is bad, however. In acute life-threatening settings, stress can be useful to create a 'fight or flight' response to get us out of dangerous situations. It is chronic or routine stress, however, that can lead to health issues such as lowered immunity, headaches, high blood pressure, heart disease, sleeplessness, anger, irritability, anxiety, and depression.

From a reproductive standpoint, stress can:

1. Alter reproductive hormones from the brain leading to problems with ovulation and implantation.
2. Increase epinephrine, which constricts blood vessels, leading to altered uterine blood flow which can adversely impact the ovaries, fallopian tubes, and uterus.

Given that everyone has stress ... the differentiating factor is that some people cope with stress more effectively or recover from stress quicker than others. The first step is to become more aware of stress. Next, consider various activities to manage your stress, such as exercise, meditation, yoga, acupuncture, massage, support groups and counseling.

Tips (From The National Institute of Mental Health)

1. Recognize signs of your body's response to stress, such as difficulty sleeping, increased alcohol and other substance use, being easily angered, feeling depressed, and having low energy.
2. Exercise regularly – 30 minutes per day of walking can boost mood and reduce stress.
3. Schedule regular times for relaxing activities (movies, hobbies, games, dining out, etc).
4. Set priorities – decide what must get done and what can wait.
5. Note what you have accomplished at the end of the day, rather than what you have not been able to do.
6. Get proper health care for existing or new health problems.
7. Stay in touch with people who can provide emotional support.
8. Ask for help from family, friends, and community or religious organizations.
9. Avoid dwelling on problems. Focusing on all the the positive things in your world.
10. Look into stress coping programs such as meditation, yoga, tai chi, massage and acupuncture.
11. If you are ever overwhelmed or in a crisis, call the toll free 24-hour National Suicide Prevention Lifeline at 1-800-273-TALK (1-800-273-8255).

Quotes

"It helps though not to get negative and down as that causes stress and doesn't help. Allow yourself to have hope--it is so important for staying positive."

•••

"Just take it one cycle at a time while always looking to the plan for the following cycle. I find it is so much easier to deal with negative pregnancy tests when you have a plan already in place for the next cycle and are always looking ahead rather than back."

• • •

"I stressed about EVERYTHING the whole pregnancy, once to the point where my husband had to take me to the ER for a panic attack. No harm came to the babies (and yes, I also stressed about my stress harming them). They're here, healthy and just turned a year old and it seems now I'll always find something to stress about with them. Just the nature of the beast I think."

• • •

"I think it helped me to move. What I mean was to exercise or do something that got out my frustrations and built up stress about infertility."

• • •

"I'm trying very hard not to obsess too much over this cycle. Or compare it to my last one. It's hard. This process is just so emotional, on its own and due to the meds."

• • •

"It is super hard not to over analyze everything. One of my favorite quotes is, 'Worry is like a rocking chair, it's something to do but it doesn't get you anywhere'."

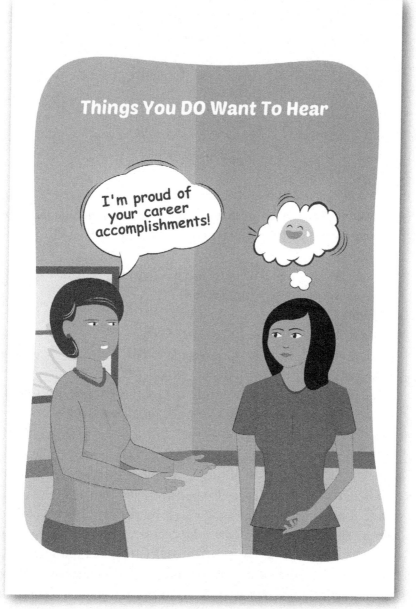

CHAPTER 36

Guilt And Anger

"Be the change you wish to see in the world."
- Mahatma Gandhi

WHEN YOU ARE not able to conceive, it is common to think that all of a sudden, everyone else but you is either pregnant or has no problem getting pregnant. It can become increasingly difficult to hear or be truly happy about things such as:

- someone else (friends / family members) being pregnant
- seeing someone else with their kids
- going to baby showers
- seeing kids in your doctor's waiting room
- being asked "when are you planning to have kids?" or "why are you waiting so long to have kids?"
- family-oriented holidays (such as Mother's Day, Father's Day, Thanksgiving, Chanukah, Christmas, or New Year's Eve)

These experiences and thoughts are quite common and, over time, can create feelings of guilt and anger. This stems from underlying feelings of helplessness and lack of control over your life plan, body, and future. We, as humans, are used to the concept of achieving our goals by planning and working hard. However, when a successful pregnancy does not occur after "working hard", it can leave you vulnerable to feeling that "life is not fair" or that you are a "failure".

Over time, guilt and anger can consume you and negatively color your everyday thoughts and experiences. Keep in mind that such feelings are a common and a normal response to infertility.

Guilt And Anger

To avoid these feelings from deepening and causing major problems, it is essential to seek fertility help early, so you can get to a successful outcome sooner. It is also important to become increasingly self-aware of such thought patterns. The next time your feel guilty or angry, ask yourself "why am I feeling this way?" Also, take a look at how your body is responding to such feelings (breathing, heart rate, tension) and the words you are using. Express your feelings or anger using sentences that begin with "I feel", rather than attacking someone who loves you.

Tips

1. Infertility is common. Many couples around you have had difficulty in getting pregnant (1 in 7) … they may have chosen not to share it with you.
2. It helps to know someone who has gone thru fertility treatments – so they can truly empathize with your journey.
3. Seek help early!
4. With proper evaluation and treatment, most all couples have a successful outcome. Everyone's journey, however, is different and can take varying amounts of time.
5. If you are feeling overwhelmed, ask your doctor for help. There are many resources including support groups and counseling.
6. Consider getting a pet.
7. Whatever feels good, do more of it. Whatever feels bad, do less.
8. Do something for someone else.
9. Talk to your clergyperson and let him/her know of your experience with infertility. They can offer a prayer and words of support for you.

Quotes

"I found out Sunday that my sister-in-law who has 2 children, the 1st one naturally a boy and the 2nd one a girl with her FIRST IVF, and now she is pregnant again after doing her FIRST IUI!!! She is 41 years old. I find that unbelievable!!! All I want is one and cannot get that. I knew that if it came out positive it would put me over the edge and it did. I cried the entire night and next day. I feel terrible that her happy news made me sad, I love her and don't want anything bad to happen, but how is one person so lucky?"

• • •

"I am the only person in my family that has ever had trouble getting pregnant. I've made a lot of progress but there are times I still get upset that my eggs went bad at a fairly young age. (late 20's-early 30's). My chances of succeeding with my eggs are very low and the chances of having a miscarriage are around 50%. I've come to the realization that the best I can do is play the hand I've been dealt, which may sound corny but helped me make peace with myself and move on to donor egg."

• • •

"I hope that I can carry a child myself. I pray on that possibility often. My sister in law just got pregnant and she was having trouble conceiving as well. A wonderful blessing but also a knife in my heart. I never let them know that. It is a joyous thing...."

Part Six

Unexpected Paths

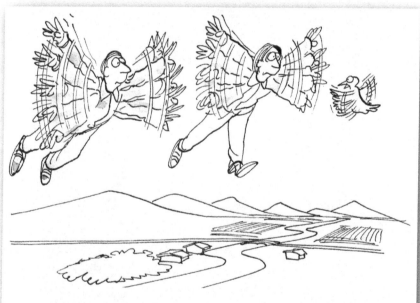

"Welcome to Change Management 101. We'll start with some free falls."

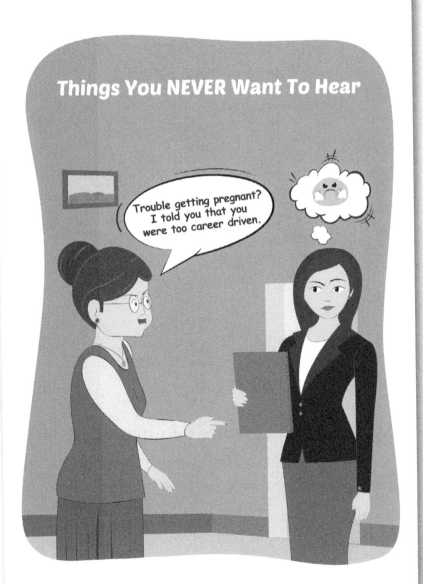

CHAPTER 37

Donor Egg

"If opportunity doesn't knock, build a door."
- Milton Berle

EGG DONATION INVOLVES use of eggs donated from another woman who is typically in her 20s or early 30s. This option takes advantage of using younger eggs, which lead to a significantly greater chance of a successful pregnancy. The first pregnancy achieved using donor eggs was in 1984. Since that time, its popularity and use has been increasing to help many couples conceive.

It is a viable and popular option for women who are typically in their 40s or for women with premature ovarian insufficiency (failure). By age 43, a woman's chance of pregnancy with IVF using her own eggs is less than 5%, and after age 45, the window is essentially closed. However, by substituting with donor eggs, the chance of pregnancy jumps to approximately 50% per attempt, regardless of patient age.

There are several methods of obtaining donor eggs:

1. Fresh anonymous donor – prospective donors can be found via agencies or IVF centers
2. Fresh known ('directed') donor – find your own prospective donor (friend, relative, via advertising)
3. Frozen donor egg bank – anonymous donor eggs already retrieved, frozen, and ready for use

In a donor egg cycle, the woman receiving the donated eggs is called the 'recipient'. By whichever method is used to obtain the donor eggs, they are fertilized in the laboratory with sperm from the recipient's partner (or a sperm donor). The recipient is given hormones to prepare her endometrium, and undergoes an embryo transfer procedure. Extra embryos can be frozen (cryopreserved) for future use. The donor egg process is also heavily regulated by the US Food and Drug Administration (FDA) to ensure treatment safety and minimize the risk of infection.

For most couples, it takes time to become comfortable with the idea of not using their own eggs. Couples will typically try treatments first with their own eggs before going with donor eggs. Complex feelings can be generated since the resulting child will be a genetic makeup of the egg donor and father, but not genetically related to the mother. It is therefore also recommended for couples considering donor eggs to meet with a counselor (social worker, psychologist) to discuss the psychosocial issues. Most fertility centers are familiar with the process and help guide patients thru this process.

Tips

1. Egg donors should preferably be between the ages of 21 and 34.
2. Recent use and experience with donor egg banks has been very promising, yielding success rates equivalent to use of fresh donor eggs.
3. All egg donors should be tested for the presence of a cystic fibrosis mutation.
4. If the recipient is over age 45, medical clearance from a primary-care doctor (including assessment of cardiac function) and maternal-fetal medicine specialist is recommended.
5. Laws may change in the future, whereby anonymity may not be guaranteed.

Donor Egg

Quotes

"We plan to tell our children where they came from as soon as they are old enough to understand. I would hope that they would feel extra special because so much was sacrificed for them...because we wanted to be parents so badly!"

• • •

"Don't rush yourself. Grieve the loss of genes for as long as you need to. And once you have had time to process everything, move forward with the excitement that you will have a baby (or more) in your arms soon!"

• • •

"I tried IVF three times without success. On our third round, our response was so poor that we had to convert the cycle to an IUI. That's when I knew it was time to move on to donor egg."

• • •

"We really just want a family- doesn't matter how we do it but I'm willing to spend the money to try with donor eggs so at least my husband will have a biological child. It doesn't seem to be that critical for him, but for some reason it's really important to me. I guess partially because I'm still feeling like I've failed him."

• • •

"I don't know how picky I am being. My family is extremely religious conservative. I don't care if they are mad at me (they are always mad at me!) but I do care about the child being ostracized. I just don't want to subject a growing child to negative feelings about how they were conceived while they are still figuring out their identity. So, long story short, I'm trying to match my looks with the donor as much as humanly possible. That's the hardest thing for me."

•••

"I chose a repeat donor. What's great is when they are a repeat donor you can look at the statistics of the previous cycles (how many days to stim, how many mature eggs received, how many fertilized, whether a pregnancy occurred, etc.). This way, you get a good gauge as to how many eggs you "may" end up with."

•••

"I tried to pick donor traits similar to me (height, hair color, etc.) but I also paid close attention to how each donor answered their questions. Some really put a lot of thought into their answers and others not so much. I was more comfortable with the donors that really put thought into their answers as I felt they would be more responsible with taking meds/adhering to appointments, etc. I don't know how much proof there is to that, but I felt the more mature the donor appeared, the more likely they would take all the prescribed meds and such."

•••

"This has been a long-drawn out process that has taken a lot of tears and self-reflection for me to reach this point. I don't regret the time I spent trying to make things work with my eggs because I needed to go through all of it so I would never look back and wonder. Just remember you have time on your side when dealing with donor eggs, so you can take plenty of time to think things through."

• • •

"I looked at the donors last night and started to cry, it all became so real. I need to get out of my funk and be happy for this opportunity."

• • •

"Something that may be of use for you to evaluate and weigh the pros and cons of donors is to do an excel spreadsheet that compares all the qualities important to you and past cycle history. Final decision is usually made by your gut, but it helps to figure out what is most important to you and when a new donor becomes available you can decide quickly if you are interested or not."

• • •

"After coming to grips that my eggs gave out on me in my early 30's is enough to make me want to go with a young donor. I know I need to look at the whole pic (like cycle history) but right now I'm focused on how my eggs started to go bad when I was still fairly young."

• • •

"When I miscarried my child created from donor egg, I grieved the same as I did with children I miscarried with my eggs. Brutal way, but effective for me to 'know' that I am ok with donor egg, whether it is my 'ideal' scenario, or anonymous, with a donor who does not share many physical or personality characteristics with me."

...

"I am sure in the end if I use an anonymous donor and carry that child to term, I will feel that it is mine 100%. It is just the uncertainty of it all. Perhaps, if I have had a child already, I would know how it felt to bond during pregnancy."

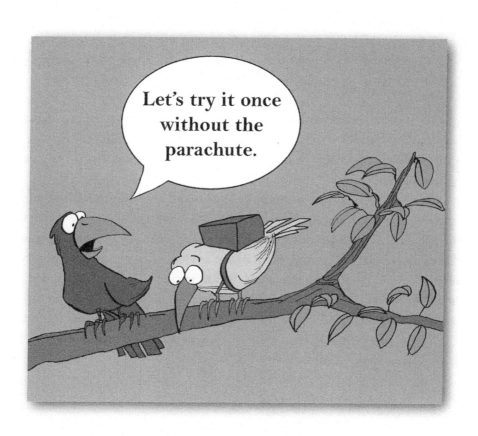

Donor Sperm

"There is no elevator to success. You have to take the stairs."
- Unknown

USE OF DONOR sperm has been long-standing, with the first reports dating back to the 1940s. Given the high prevalence of male-factor infertility as well as increasing use by single women and same-sex couples, it remains a popular option for many to build their families.

There are several donor sperm banks around the country that obtain, freeze, store and sell frozen sperm. The sperm donation process is regulated by the Food and Drug Administration (FDA) to minimize any infectious disease risk to the recipient. Potential sperm donors undergo a comprehensive history, physical examination, and infectious disease testing at time of sperm donation. The sperm is then quarantined for at least six months at which time the donor is re-tested for infectious diseases, before the sperm is released for use.

Sperm donors should be at least 18 years of age and preferably under 40 years. Donor sperm can be obtained by:

1. Anonymous sperm donors
   o Via sperm banks as noted above.
2. Known (directed) donors
   o The FDA exempts known donors from the six-month re-testing requirement, but ASRM recommends it be done.

There are two types of samples offered by most sperm banks: intracervical insemination (ICI) and intrauterine insemination (IUI) specimens. ICI specimens must be washed/prepared for IUI, whereas IUI specimens are pre-washed. Most fertility centers have the ability to prepare/wash sperm specimens – thereby allowing you to obtain the less-expensive ICI specimens.

Once donor sperm via a sperm bank is selected and paid for, the sperm bank ships the vial(s) of frozen sperm in special containers to your fertility center. The fertility center takes these frozen vials and keeps them frozen till you are ready for your procedure. Typically, one vial is used per IUI or IVF procedure.

Complex feelings can be generated since the resulting child will be a genetic makeup of the sperm donor and mother, but not genetically related to the father. It is therefore also recommended for couples considering donor sperm to meet with a counselor (social worker, psychologist) to discuss the psychosocial issues. Most fertility centers are familiar with the process and help guide patients thru this process.

Tips

1. Sperm banks provide pictures of the donor as well as detailed information about their education, hobbies, and interests.
2. Ask your fertility center if you can purchase the less-expensive ICI sperm specimens.
3. A positive CMV result from a sperm donor does not make the donor ineligible, since his sperm can be used with CMV-positive recipients.
4. Laws may change in the future, whereby anonymity may not be guaranteed.

Quotes

"My husband was very reluctant to just pick the donors on his own and never looked at the information on the internet. I printed out all the info and showed it to him and then we listened to the donor interview on line and made our choice."

•••

"It is hard for some men to come to the realization that they cannot father a child."

•••

"My husband wanted nothing to do with the whole process. Didn't want a donor, then didn't want to have a kid ever know they came from a donor, then changed his mind again. And did a little back and forth on the whole thing. It took a year for him to finally come around. We did the final choosing together."

•••

"I won't say there aren't times were he tells me it is hard for him because he is not the 'biological' father- he knows that being the sperm giver does not make someone a DAD! There are so many deadbeat dads out there that were actually nothing more than a sperm donor. He is right biologically he is not their father. But he is more of a dad than anyone could possibly be. Sometimes I feel he tries even harder to be the best possible dad. Donor sperm is not for everyone, but if you find a way to separate the genetic piece - It is your BABY, no one else's! It's the whole argument of nature vs nurture."

•••

"My husband glows every time people say the kids look like him, and he's crazy about our babies, even if they don't have his genes."

CHAPTER 39

Donor Embryos

"If we believe that tomorrow will be better, we can bear a hardship today."
- Thich Nhat Hanh

EMBRYO DONATION IS a process that allows embryos that were created by couples undergoing IVF treatment to be used by other infertile patients to achieve a pregnancy. It is also sometimes referred to as 'embryo adoption'. It is estimated that there are over 600,000 frozen embryos in storage in the United States.

Similar to use of donor eggs/sperm, the embryo donor process is also regulated by the FDA (to minimize risk of infectious disease transmission). For previously created embryos, the FDA recommends, but does not require, that the couple who created these embryos undergo the requisite screening and testing required of all egg and sperm donors. If embryos are being created solely for donation, the egg and sperm donors must be screened and tested for infectious diseases.

Embryo donation is relatively less common than use of donor eggs and sperm, since many infertile couples have a difficult time giving up their frozen embryos for donation. The chance of pregnancy from donor embryos depends on the age of the female who provided the eggs as well as the quality of the embryos.

Tips

1. Use of donor embryos is appealing to couples that may need donor eggs, in part due to its relatively lower cost.

2. Besides individual fertility centers, there are several agencies that provide access to donor embryos.
3. Many fertility centers have embryo donation programs that assist you with the legal agreements.

Quotes

"We decided on donated embryos. It didn't matter to us if the babies were genetically linked to me or my husband, so we went for it. I looked at it this way ... a 10% chance with my own eggs, (basically throwing money out the window for a very small chance) or a 50% chance of success with our donated embryos. Also, it was much cheaper, so we could do a heck of a lot of transfers for even half the cost of donor eggs or another IVF cycle using my crappy eggs. I have never regretted our choice one. These babies are mine in every way possible!"

• • •

"It helped me to cope with the stress of our last cycle by discovering donor embryos. It is so much cheaper than IVF. It is an FET only."

• • •

"We suffered from three miscarriages before finally having our little boy. After the second miscarriage, we decided to go to donor embryos. My hubby was a lot happier with using donor embryos than sperm for some reason. I think he wanted to feel like we had the same relationship to the child. I was fine either way. It was the best decision we could have made!"

CHAPTER 40

Gestational Carrier

*"Always bear in mind that your own resolution to succeed is
more important than any other."*
- Abraham Lincoln

GESTATIONAL CARRIERS (GC; also called 'gestational surrogates') are
women who agree to carry a pregnancy created by transferring an embryo
created with the sperm and egg of the intended parents. Of note, donor eggs
and/or donor sperm may also be used. It is a complex process that requires
careful coordination by medical professionals, lawyers, and mental health
professionals.

A GC is used when a true medical condition prevents the intended parent
from carrying a pregnancy or would pose a significant risk of death or harm to
the woman or the fetus. Examples of such medical indications include:

- Significant uterine abnormality
- Absence of uterus
- Medical contraindication to pregnancy (e.g., pulmonary hyperten-
  sion, heart failure)
- Serious medical condition that could worsen with pregnancy or harm
  the fetus

A GC may also be considered for women who have a history that suggests a problem with her endometrial lining (such as recurrent miscarriage
or multiple IVF failures), or when a female partner is absent (single male or
gay couple).

A GC should ideally have the following characteristics:

- healthy and between the ages of 21 and 45
- have had at least one successful term pregnancy
- have no more than five previous vaginal deliveries or two prior cesarean deliveries
- have a supportive family environment

The GC undergoes a complete history and physical exam, as well as comprehensive lab testing for infectious diseases (including HIV, gonorrhea, chlamydia, hepatitis, syphilis, and CMV). The GC and her partner typically also undergo an interview/evaluation with a qualified mental health professional. This process covers the psychological risks associated with being a GC.

Similar to the GC, the intended parents also undergo the history, physical exam, and lab testing. Counseling with a mental health professional is also encouraged for the intended parents. The evaluation will cover, in part, the couple's relationship and expectations with the GC and her family, plans for any relationship with the GC after delivery, and plans to disclose the use of a GC to the child that is born.

In the United States, every state has its own laws (or lack thereof) governing use of GCs. It is important that the intended parents and GC retain independent reproductive lawyers who are knowledgeable with GC laws and contracts in the states where the parties live, intend to receive Ob care, and intend to deliver. A typical GC-intended parent contract may include agreements on compensation to the GC, number of embryos to transfer, testing to be done during pregnancy, and contingent plans in the event of multiple pregnancies or the presence of fetal anomalies.

Tips

1. Use of GC in the United States is relatively infrequent and expensive (the cost can range from $60,000 - $120,000+).

2. Seek a fertility center with experience using GCs. They can walk you thru the complex process.
3. There are many agencies that can help find suitable GCs.
4. Learn about the GC laws in your state.

CHAPTER 41

Adoption

"Happiness is a journey, not a destination."
- Ben Sweetland

FOR COUPLES STRUGGLING with infertility, the decision to move to adoption does not come easy. Most couples want to experience a pregnancy and have a child with at least some of their genetics. However, for some couples, adoption is the right path towards achieving parenthood.

There are many different pathways and types of adoption, each with different procedures and requirements (domestic vs international vs foster care). Adoptions can be arranged via a private, county, or state agency, or independently (either domestic or international).

Almost all US private adoptions are of very young babies, with many newborns going home from the hospital with their adoptive parents. In contrast, for international adoptions in 2013, 8% of children adopted were younger than 1-year-old, 54% were 1-4 years, and 38% were older than 4 years. Also, the majority of children adopted internationally are Asian, African, or Latin American (less than 15% are Caucasian). Children adopted from foster care range in age from infants to 17 years (average age is 8) … with 24% African American, 42% Caucasian, and 23% Hispanic.

In the US, every state has different laws on adoption. Furthermore, every country has its own rules and regulations. If you decide to go international, begin to learn the laws, policies, and cultural issues of that specific country. Parent age requirements vary by country. Most countries require parents to be between the ages of 25 and 50, though some have younger cutoffs.

Adoptions are also classified as 'closed' or 'open'. Closed adoptions don't provide information on the birth parents and less common today. Most domestic adoptions are open, meaning the birth parents and the adoptive parents share identifying information. In international adoptions, there has traditionally been little to no contact with the child's birth parents, but this is changing to a more open system.

Adoption can also be an expensive process, with costs ranging from $20,000 to $60,000. Foster care adoptions tend to be significantly less expensive, often with minimal cost. International adoptions also incur significant travel, food, and lodging costs (as well as time off work). The Internal Revenue Service (IRS) does provide an adoption expense federal tax credit (up to $13,400 for tax year 2015) based on type of adoption and income (www.irs.gov/taxtopics/tc607.html).

Wait times for adoption can vary widely depending on where the child is from and other characteristics (e.g., race/ethnicity, special needs). A basic timeline for adoption can look like the following:

1. 1-3 months – learn about adoption; attend information session; make initial decision about type of adoption.
2. 3-6 months – choose adoption agency and attorney; begin locating your child.
3. 6-9 months – complete home study (visit to your home by a social worker to verify you are able to care for a child); collect relevant documents (birth/marriage certificates, references, tax returns); begin adoption process.
4. 9-24 months – receive match with expectant mother (domestic) or child referral (international)
5. 12-30 months – birth of baby or placement of child to you → success!
6. 18-36 months – finalization of adoption (post-placement reports, final court hearing)

Tips

1. Gathering information is essential. Conduct a lot of research and talk to other parents who have successfully adopted children.
2. Learn the laws and regulations early.

3. Some couples begin the adoption process while they are undergoing fertility treatment. Do what feels right for you.
4. Regardless of the type of adoption you choose, it can be a very rewarding experience.

Quotes

"I feel like I have put so much physical and emotional energy into overcoming infertility that I just don't know if I have it in me to deal with the process of donor/adoption."

● ● ●

"We adopted our son. He is now 2 years old. We were able to see him shortly after he was born and able to bring him home from the hospital and now 2 years later can't imagine NOT having him in our family!"

● ● ●

"I am 38 and my husband is 39. I was officially diagnosed with PCOS. I have suspected it for some time, but could not get my Gyn to diagnose. I finally changed Gyns and my new Gyn immediately sent me to an RE who found we also had male infertility issues. Before starting treatment, we moved to a very rural area 6+ hours from any specialist and just could not find a way to get treatment. So we adopted two beautiful girls."

● ● ●

Adoption

"My husband and I have been trying to conceive for 9 years. I was diagnosed with PCOS 6 years ago. I have gone through all the various treatments with limited success (3 miscarriages). I am 33 and my husband is 34. We are taking a two-year hiatus on trying to conceive, and are working on an adoption plan."

•••

"For us 8 years of putting our marriage on a calendar without spontaneity and focused on a baby made me lose myself and us lose sight of why we fell in love. We decided in September, we did all we could, now we just wanted a family and a marriage. So, we are pursuing adoption and taking a break from infertility, maybe permanently, we will see. But for now, I am trusting in God that I should have a family anyway he wants to give it to me. This journey takes a lot of soul searching, and challenging times, but the good news is we can all come out of it winners."

Part Seven

Outcomes

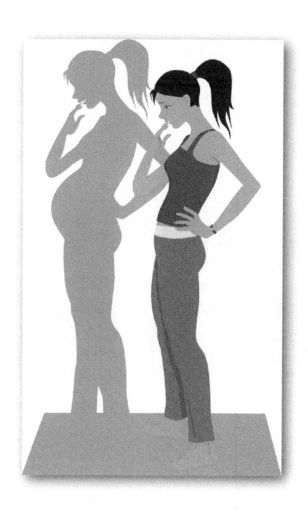

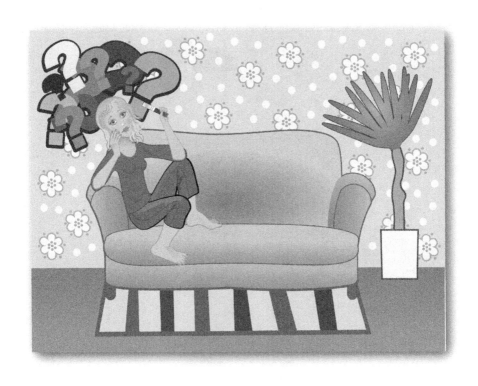

CHAPTER 42

Not Pregnant

"I've failed over and over and over again in my life, and that is why I succeed."
- Michael Jordan

AS MUCH AS everyone is cheering for you to have a positive outcome, you must be prepared for the dreaded call telling you that your treatment cycle was not successful. Unfortunately, there are no guarantees or sure things in the area of reproduction. We can blame 'nature' or a 'higher-power' for setting up such an imperfect system.

It is important to also know that most couples that have patience and persistence go on to have a successful pregnancy. Therefore, it is helpful to set realistic expectations when beginning your fertility journey. Know that it will take time and there may be some ups and downs along the way. Many couples go thru this process … and with proper support and a good medical team … you WILL eventually have success!

Tips

1. Before starting treatment, ask your doctor what the realistic chances are for your treatment to lead to a pregnancy and live birth.
2. Avoid comparing your chances to other people you know who have undergone fertility treatment. Every couple has different circumstances and medical factors that impact their outcomes.

3. Have a next step/treatment plan already worked out before finding out the results of your pregnancy test. Your fertility nurse/doctor can help you with this.
4. Have a support system around you (spouse, relatives, friends) when you hear the news of a negative pregnancy test. It helps to have a shoulder to lean on.
5. Hang in there. You are not alone. You WILL eventually have success!

Quotes

"I had given up so many times and after each failed one my heart hurt a little more. It took all I had to do it a 4th time and thank God I did."

• • •

"The numbness and disappointment is hard to deal with month by month. I had a bfn negative this cycle and thought I was for sure pregnant, so I know what you are going through. No matter what, the sadness is there and its best to try to process it pick yourself up and try again. Instead of trying to hold it all in, I let myself feel all the emotions that come with infertility like anger, jealously, sadness, and emptiness. However, I always remind myself that there is next month to look forward too and to stay positive for the next round then to stay stuck in the disappointment that this round wasn't successful."

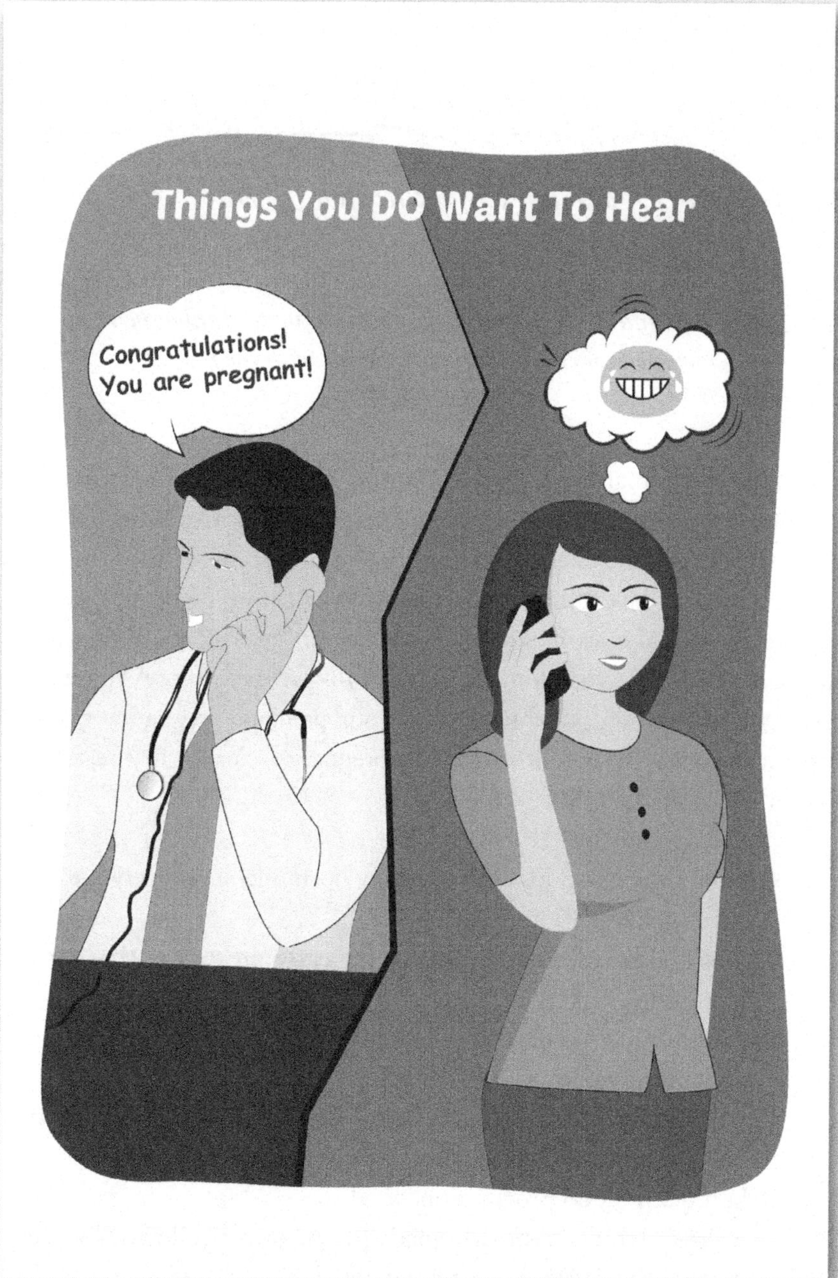
Things You DO Want To Hear
Congratulations! You are pregnant!

CHAPTER 43

Positive Pregnancy Test!

"The best and most beautiful things in the world cannot be seen or even touched. They must be felt with the heart."
- Helen Keller

AFTER RUNNING A marathon, there is nothing more exhilarating than crossing the finish line. Hearing that your pregnancy test is positive for the first time will likely feel similar. All the effort you have put in seems to have finally paid off! You will likely be calling you partner to share the excitement as well.

After the initial elation, you may start becoming a bit cautious, knowing that the next phase of your journey is beginning ... pregnancy! You will now want to do everything possible to keep your precious pregnancy safe. Your fertility center will start following your pregnancy closely, in the following manner:

1. Follow your blood hCG (pregnancy hormone) level every 2 to 3 days till it gets above 1500 mIU/ml
   o hCG is made by the cells of the early pregnancy that form the placenta.
   o A minimal increase in hCG is 35% in 48 hours for a potentially viable pregnancy.
   o A suboptimal increase in hCG could signify a possible miscarriage or ectopic pregnancy.
2. Check your blood progesterone level
   o Progesterone is initially made by the ovary, followed by the placenta (by 8-10 weeks of pregnancy).

- Since progesterone is released in a pulsatile manner, it can often vary significantly during the course of a day.
- The optimal progesterone level is controversial, but most fertility centers are reassured by a level at or above 15-20 ng/ml.
3. Perform several transvaginal ultrasounds
   - First ultrasound done at about 6 weeks of pregnancy or when hCG level>1500 mIU/ml. In a normal pregnancy, we should see a clear 'gestational sac' (round structure) in the uterus by 6 weeks.
   - Absence of a gestational sac is concerning for a miscarriage or ectopic pregnancy
   - Ultrasound at 7 weeks of pregnancy should show a clear fetus (also called a 'fetal pole') measuring about 1 cm with a heartbeat (typically over 100 beats per minute).
   - Ultrasound by 9-10 weeks of pregnancy should show a fetus measuring about 2-3 cm with a heart rate of 170-180 bpm. Also, fetal movement may be seen!

With everything going well, by about 10-12 weeks of pregnancy, most fertility centers will refer you back to your Ob/Gyn who will continue taking care of your pregnancy. If you are also on estrogen and/or progesterone supplementation, you will be weaned off these supplements by this time.

Tips

1. The time period after your IUI (intrauterine insemination) or embryo transfer is often called the *two-week wait* (2WW). It is considered by many patients to be a most challenging time of waiting. Consider the following during this time:
2. Do not do a home pregnancy test. It can often be falsely positive, because the hCG 'trigger' shot can give the test a false reading.
3. Avoid minimizing your activity during this time, since it is not helpful. Try to lead your normal day-to-day routine. Do not start a new exercise routine during this time.

4. Avoid lifting heavy objects, doing strenuous work, or using saunas, steam rooms, and hot tubs.
5. Don't stop taking your medications till you do your blood pregnancy test as scheduled.
6. Avoid travelling (especially by air) until your pregnancy is confirmed to be in the uterus.
7. An hCG level that rises very quickly can signify a possible twin or triplet pregnancy.
8. An early twin pregnancy on initial ultrasound can sometimes self-reduce to a single pregnancy within the first 12 weeks ('vanishing twin syndrome'). Therefore, wait until 12 weeks before telling others you are having twins.

Quotes

"I know it's easy to say not to worry and to enjoy every minute of being pregnant, but with each pregnancy I've tried to follow the idea of not worrying until someone told me to (or until something like spotting made me think I should)."

•••

"It's totally normal to worry. I've been obsessed about every little pain I felt and those statistics about miscarriage during my first trimester. I think once you enter the second trimester, you will be somewhat relieved and finally get to believe that you are going to be mom and enjoy the pregnancy!"

•••

"I was fearful till I was holding her in my arms...I had a rough pregnancy with bed rest and several issues, but I know several women who have had IVF and were terrified whole pregnancy. I freaked over every little thing...but sometimes it was good I was so in tune too."

•••

"I enjoy my pregnancy as much as possible but worry a lot of the time. With every milestone you hit hopefully you will get a bit more comfortable and confident."

•••

"I wanted to relax and just assume the best was going to happen. But I worried and fretted and was a basket case before every ultrasound and doctor's appointment. I did manage to also give myself permission to enjoy the wonder and savor the experience. Eventually."

•••

"There is always hope! Fortunately, I've had some great news recently... I am pregnant! Our first cycle using injectables (and IUI) did the trick. I am struggling with being able to let myself get excited and don't really know how to let go of all my fears/worry about these early weeks."

•••

"It's a daily struggle for me to give over my worries to God and ask Him to take care of me and this tiny life inside of me. I go for my 2nd ultrasound on Monday (I'll be 6 weeks) and I'm still debating telling our families the news on Mother's Day."

•••

"It's hard to wait to tell family as soon as you are pregnant, I couldn't the first time. But next time I may be a little gun shy and might wait to tell them until I pass the 12-week point. Oh who am I kidding, I will tell my mom and sister the day I find out probably."

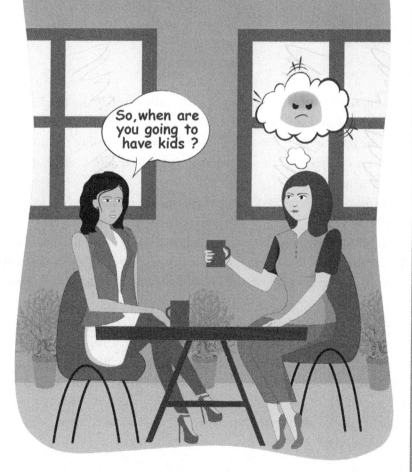

CHAPTER 44

Miscarriage / Recurrent Pregnancy Loss

"Life affords no higher pleasure than that of surmounting difficulties."
-Samuel Johnson

A MISCARRIAGE (SPONTANEOUS abortion) is unfortunately the most common complication of an early pregnancy. It occurs quite frequently, regardless of whether the pregnancy is conceived naturally or thru fertility treatment. It is a traumatic experience for the couple, especially when a lot of effort went into achieving the pregnancy.

The miscarriage rate is dependent on the age of the mother, as follows: age 20-30 (11-15%); age 35 (20-25%); age 40 (40-50%); age 45 (80-90%). The increasing miscarriage risk associated with increasing maternal age is related to the progressive decline in egg quality with age. The chance of a miscarriage decreases as a pregnancy advances, as follows:<6 weeks (22-57%); 6-10 weeks (15%);>10 weeks (3-5%).

The most common cause of a miscarriage is due to spontaneous chromosomal (genetic) abnormalities in the embryo (e.g., aneuploidy, mosaicism, translocation, inversion, deletion). These account for 50-60% of all miscarriages. Most such abnormalities occur spontaneously and are not inherited from a parent.

The following additional lifestyle factors are associated with an increased risk of miscarriage:

- Heavy smoking (>10 cigarettes per day) --- 3x increased risk
- Consuming>3 alcohol drinks per week
- Cocaine use

- Use of NSAIDs (ibuprofen) around the time of conception
- Very high doses of caffeine (1000mg or 10 cups of coffee per day)
- Pre-pregnancy body-mass index (BMI)<18.5 or above 25 kg/m^2
- Fever>100°F (27.8°C)

As difficult as one pregnancy loss may be, some women have to face dealing with consecutive pregnancy losses … also known as 'recurrent pregnancy loss (RPL)'. The medical definition of RPL has evolved over the years, with ASRM defining it as: two or more failed *clinical* pregnancies. It is important to note that a 'clinical' pregnancy requires being able to visualize it via transvaginal ultrasound. Therefore, a very early pregnancy loss before it can be seen via ultrasound (biochemical pregnancy) does not meet the criteria.

RPL is relatively uncommon, with about 2% of women experiencing two consecutive pregnancy losses, and about 0.4-1% having three consecutive losses. A woman with two prior losses has a recurrence risk of about 25%, 30% after 3 losses, and 40% after four losses. RPL is certainly an extremely traumatic experience for couples, and is associated with high rates of severe stress and depression.

A comprehensive evaluation will identify at least one cause in about 50-60% of couples. The known causes of RPL can be categorized as follows:

1. Genetic (3-5%)
   - About 3-5% of RPL couples have an abnormality in their chromosomes (versus 0.7% of the general population). It is 3 times more common in women.
   - Recommended testing: blood test for man and woman called *karyotype*.
   - The most common finding is called a '*balanced translocation*' – where portions of two chromosomes are exchanged, without loss of chromosome function. However, if these genes are inherited in an unbalanced way, it can cause a pregnancy loss. There are commonly two types of such translocations:
     - Reciprocal translocation (60%)
       - When two chromosome break and exchange material; parent still has 46 total chromosomes.

- Leads to 10-15% risk of having a child with a major birth defect.
    - Robertsonian translocation (40%)
        - When two chromosomes combine; parent therefore has 45 total chromosomes.
        - Commonly involve chromosomes 13, 14, 15, 21, or 22; a combination between chromosome 14 and 21 is considered most relevant.
        - If mother has the translocation → 10-15% risk of an abnormal child.
        - If father has the translocation → 0-2% risk of an abnormal child.
2. Uterine abnormalities (20%)
    - may be present from birth (congenital) or acquired later in life.
    - Recommended test: saline-infusion ultrasound (sonoHSG), hysteroscopy, and/or hysterosalpingogram (HSG).
    - Abnormalities include:
        a. Fibroids
            - The type that protrude into the uterine cavity (submucous fibroids) can prevent a pregnancy or increase the risk of miscarriage.
        b. Endometrial polyps
        c. Septate uterus
            - If present, can increase the risk of miscarriage to 60-80%.
            - The longer the septum, the higher the miscarriage risk.
        d. Intrauterine adhesions (scar tissue; also known as 'Asherman Syndrome')
            - There is an increased risk of scar tissue formation inside the uterus after a D&C procedure (especially after giving birth).
3. Immunologic factors (5-15%)
    - Presence of antibodies in the blood that can increase the risk of forming blood clots in the placenta.

- Recommended blood tests: Anticardiolipin antibodies (IgG & IgM), lupus anticoagulant, anti-beta2-glycoprotein antibodies (IgG & IgM).
- If initial test is positive, the test should be repeated after at least 12 weeks to confirm presence.
- Recommended treatment: baby aspirin and heparin

4. Endocrine (hormonal) abnormalities (15-20%)
    - Recommended blood tests: TSH, free T4, Prolactin, day 3 FSH & Estradiol, AMH.
    - Progesterone is required for successful implantation and maintenance of pregnancy. The presence of abnormal progesterone production ('luteal phase defect'), however, is controversial. Furthermore, progesterone blood levels frequently vary with the same day and are of limited value.
    - Adding routine progesterone supplementation in the luteal phase (prior to pregnancy establishment) may be beneficial to prevent a future miscarriage.
    - Possible causes:
        a. Hypothyroidism (underactive thyroid)
            - Goal of treatment is a TSH between 1.0 and 2.5 mIU/mL.
        b. Hyperprolactinemia (high prolactin)
        c. Uncontrolled diabetes
        d. Obesity
        e. Decreased ovarian reserve

5. Psychological factors
    - RPL invokes significant emotional distress, often leading to increased anxiety, anger, guilt, grief, and depression.
    - Small studies indicate that with adequate psychological counseling/support and close monitoring, patients have a lower chance of a subsequent miscarriage.

6. Unexplained (40-50%)
    - This can be extremely frustrating for couples, since most want to find a cause that can be 'fixed'. It is common to have feelings of anger toward your medical team for 'not having an answer'.

Outcomes

- ○ Progesterone supplementation may be beneficial in such circumstances.
- ○ 60-70% of women with unexplained RPL go on to have a successful next pregnancy.

Tips

1. Exercise, intercourse, and dietary indulgences do not cause a miscarriage. Do not blame yourself.
2. The grief reaction after a miscarriage can often be similar to that associated with the death of an adult.
3. If you are experiencing a miscarriage, as your doctor if the failed pregnancy tissue can be tested for chromosome abnormalities (karyotype testing).
4. Oral progesterone is not as effective as vaginal or intramuscular progesterone.
5. Routine use of a baby aspirin, heparin, or steroids (prednisone) does not prevent a miscarriage, and may lead to other complications.
6. Over 20 high-quality clinical trials confirm there is no benefit of immunotherapy to prevent a miscarriage.
7. Routine endometrial biopsy for dating the endometrium is unreliable and not recommended.
8. To date, no infectious agents have been found to increase the risk of miscarriages. Routine use of antibiotics is therefore not recommended.
9. Routine use of sperm for DNA fragmentation is not recommended, since such testing is not correlated with RPL.

Quotes

"It was the happiest moment when I found out I was pregnant for the 1st time (1st IUI) in my life. It's one of those things that I wish I could hang on to forever, but so sad it's just so short. My hCG dropped at 6 weeks and was told this could an abnormal pregnancy. I haven't stopped crying since."

●●●

"After 4 IUIs we finally got our cherished positive hCG only for it to end in a miscarriage at 8 weeks ... after taking couple months off I'm now waiting for my period to start so that we can do another IUI ... we got the RPL back with nothing wrong ... my husband and the RE are very optimistic that I'll get pregnant again this IUI since we will be using the same protocol as last time. I'm afraid to even get optimistic about it since I'm so scared it will take another year before we see any results … I don't know why, but I'm so so nervous and scared ... I dread getting another short lived positive hCG and I also dread getting no positive hCG ... I'm upset still every Monday which used to mark another week of pregnancy for me ... but I also get upset at sitting idle and not trying ... I don't know what to do ... these last few months have transformed me into a different person. I used to be happy and carefree and now I'm never content, resentful and mostly just angry all the time."

●●●

"How do I get the courage to start this journey over? Those of you who have suffered loss and have tried again, please help me understand."

●●●

"It is hard to cycle after a miscarriage, I was worried the entire time about another miscarriage or a negative test, but I was successful our next cycle after it and went on to have a healthy pregnancy."

●●●

"I had a cousin tell me after a loss few years ago, "Just get over it! You weren't even that far along!" I haven't spoken to him since."

• • •

"I'm scared...I'm absolutely terrified of another loss. However, I am more afraid of not having another child and the only way to get to a place where I can have a baby is to do all of the emotional gymnastics that come with TTC. I just have to trust that if it's meant to happen, it will. If it doesn't, or if we have another loss, then at least I tried all I could."

• • •

"After my early loss, I didn't want to go thru another cycle. I did it for my husband, and went into it expecting it not to work, and it didn't. After that we took a vacation and it really helped us both refocus and realize there's more to life than fertility treatments. It was good to have that week away full of distractions and fun things. When we came back, I was in a much better frame of mind and approached my next cycle with a positive attitude. I went into it confident that it would work, and it did!"

• • •

"I did not even do a baby shower because I was scared I would jinx the pregnancy (and I was totally aware this was nuts). I was terrified of miscarrying again. and I would love to say I have loosened up on this pregnancy--but honestly, until that baby is in my arms I won't breath totally easy."

• • •

"Grief is a process with many stages and there are no timelines as to when we hit those stages. Each person is so different. I still have times I struggle with my losses."

• • •

"I don't think the ache over lost babies every completely goes away, but the sharpness of the pain does dull over time. I also find the bad days are fewer and farther between than they were in that first month or two. There is no set amount of time to heal emotionally after a miscarriage. The timer won't go off at three months past and we'll suddenly be all better. We won't ever not grieve the loss or not wonder what might have been, and the "normal" we return to after the immediate pain of the loss subsides is a new normal so we grieve who we were before the loss a bit too. It's still hard for me to get over the fact that we almost got what we hoped for and that there's no guarantee that it will actually work in the future. Seems like a cruel tease to get that close. It was particularly hard when those who got pregnant around the same time as me had their babies. It was hard when my due date came and went. It's hard seeing others sporting baby bumps that are about the same size as mine should be."

• • •

"I had IVF last year and miscarried at 9 weeks. Thank goodness we decided to do a testing on the fetus and it came back positive for Trisomy 14. We then did testing on both of us and that's how we realized that my husband has a Robertsonian Translocation."

• • •

"I have been irregular for as long as I can remember. I saw multiple different Gynecologists and they put me on the pill each time trying something different because they made me crazy! About 2 years ago my husband and I decided to start trying to get pregnant. I knew it was going to be a challenge, but little did we know it was going to test us to the limits. Finally, after 6 months, they started doing all of the infertility testing and found nothing. So, I went on Clomid®. I was fortunate to get pregnant on the first try. But, by week 9 I miscarried and we found out it was blighted ovum. About 2 months later, I got pregnant on my own. Within a week of the positive test, I miscarried (chemical pregnancy). Well, not planning, we got pregnant the next month. Everything was going great until at 22 weeks we went in for a routine ultrasound and she had no heartbeat. It was devastating. We are not giving up and will be seeing an RE to help us."

CHAPTER 45

Ectopic Pregnancy

"Failure will never overtake me if my determination to succeed is strong enough."
- Og Mandino

AN ECTOPIC PREGNANCY is the consequence of an embryo implanting outside of the uterus. It occurs in 1-2% of all pregnancies and is always abnormal. The diagnosis is usually unexpected and emotionally traumatic. It is additionally challenging because once the diagnosis is made, it requires expedient medical or surgical treatment so that it does not become life threatening.

The most common location of the ectopic pregnancy is the fallopian tube (98%), but they can also occur in the ovary, cervix, or abdomen. There is currently no surgical way to remove and transplant the ectopic pregnancy into the uterus. A rare form of ectopic pregnancy is called 'heterotopic pregnancy' – this is when there is an ectopic pregnancy along with an intrauterine pregnancy. It is more common among couples undergoing IVF.

Women who have a history of tubal disease/damage are at higher risk for ectopics. Causes of tubal disease include infections (gonorrhea, chlamydia), endometriosis, appendicitis, or prior surgery. Women who have had a prior ectopic are 10-15x more likely to have a second ectopic pregnancy.

The most common clinical presentation of an ectopic pregnancy is vaginal bleeding and/or abdominal pain, which typically appear 6-8 weeks after the last normal menstrual period. Among patients who conceive via fertility treatments, they are most often followed very closely from the beginning of their pregnancy. If their blood hCG levels are not rising appropriately, an ectopic pregnancy gets suspected early, prior to the onset of any symptoms. This early suspicion fortunately leads to an early diagnosis, often before the onset of symptoms.

The combination of blood hCG levels and trans-vaginal ultrasound lead to the diagnosis of ectopics. When the hCG level reaches 1500 mIU/mL, a pregnancy (gestational sac) should be visualized in the uterus (also see Chapter on 'Positive Pregnancy Test'). If not present, then there is significant concern for a possible ectopic pregnancy. It is also possible that it could be a failed intrauterine pregnancy. Close follow up with your doctor every 2-3 days will help solidify the diagnosis. Sometimes, if no clear ectopic is seen but the pregnancy is clearly abnormal – the diagnosis of 'presumed ectopic' is made in order to initiate timely treatment.

There are two main ways to treat ectopic pregnancies:

1. Medical
   o Among patients who underwent fertility treatment, most ectopic pregnancies are successfully treated medically using a medication called Methotrexate (MTX). MTX was originally developed to treat cancer cells, but was later found to also be effective in dissolving ectopic pregnancies.
   o The overall success rate of MTX treatment is about 90%.
   o The ideal candidates have an hCG level<5000 mIU/mL and ectopic size<4 cm with no fetal cardiac activity.
   o MTX is given as an intramuscular injection followed by close monitoring of your hCG levels to make sure they start going down appropriately.
   o 85% of patients may have a transient increase in hCG levels, before seeing a decline.
   o 20% of patients may need a second dose of MTX.
   o The average resolution time is 35 days.
   o Once starting MTX treatment the following instructions are important:
     ▪ no alcohol intake
     ▪ stop prenatal vitamins and folic acid
     ▪ no intercourse / sexual activity

- avoid prolonged sun exposure and gas-producing foods (beans, leeks, cabbage)
- do not use aspirin or ibuprofen
- do not travel till the ectopic is resolved

2. Surgical
   - Surgery is necessary for the following reasons: internal bleeding; clinical signs of impending ectopic rupture; MTX not an option or has failed.
   - Most surgeries are accomplished via laparoscopy under general anesthesia. If the ectopic has not ruptured, an attempt is made to remove the ectopic from the tube ('linear salpingostomy'). However, if the tube is rupture, damaged, or bleeding significantly, it is removed ('salpingectomy').
   - An overnight hospital stay is usually not necessary after the laparoscopy.
   - After surgery, it is important to have close follow up to ensure your hCG level returns back to zero.

Tips

1. Smoking increases the risk of ectopics in a dose-dependent manner – the more you smoke, the higher the risk.
2. Ectopic pregnancy may also occur after IVF treatment (1-2% of the time).
3. Women with an ectopic who have a baseline hCG>5000 mIU/mL are more likely to need multiple doses of MTX or experience treatment failure.
4. Mild abdominal pain of short duration (1-2 days) may occur a week after starting MTX therapy.
5. Treatment with MTX does not compromise ovarian reserve.
6. The risk of another ectopic pregnancy is the same for both medical and surgical therapies.

7. There is no known deleterious effect of previous MTX treatment on future pregnancies. Patients may attempt to conceive again once their hCG levels are back to zero.

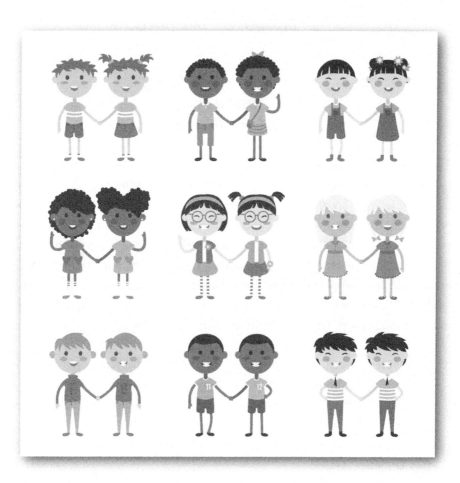

CHAPTER 46

Multiple Pregnancy

"Nothing is IMPOSSIBLE, the word itself says, I'M POSSIBLE!"
- Audrey Hepburn

THE RISK OF multiple pregnancy (e.g. twins, triplets) has been increasing over the past decades, largely due to increasing use of fertility treatments. With improved technology and use of treatment guidelines, the majority of multiple pregnancies from treatment tend to be twins. The goal of fertility centers, however, is to optimize the chances of a patient delivering a single, healthy child.

It is quite common for many infertility patients to want twins, since it may result in a completed family from one treatment/pregnancy. It is the job of the medical team, however, to educate patients about the risks of having a multiple pregnancy. They can be summarized as follows:

1. Preterm birth – 57% of twins, 93% of triplets; prematurity can lead to significant health problems (respiratory disease, bowel damage, eye damage, bleeding in brain, cerebral palsy), learning disabilities, and physical handicaps.
2. Very low birth weight infants (<1500 grams) – 10% of twins, 37% of triplets
3. Born before 32 weeks – 11% of twins, 41% of triplets
4. Birth defects
5. Placental abnormalities – leading to abnormal fetal growth and development
6. Fetal death – 5.5 per 1000 in single births; 24 per 1000 for twins; 55 per 1000 for triplets

7. Admission to neonatal intensive care unit (NICU) – 25% of twins, 75% of triplets
7. Maternal risks – increased risks of bleeding, miscarriage, diabetes, preeclampsia, liver disease, blood clots, chronic back pain. Women are 6x more likely to be hospitalized with pregnancy complications.
8. Psychosocial issues following birth – severe parenting stress, parental depression, child abuse, and divorce.
9. Economic implications – higher costs to care for children, increased costs from potential child disabilities, need for extra caregivers, and time off from work.

The greater the number of fetuses within the uterus, the greater is the risk for adverse outcomes. Patients who do have a pregnancy with more than twins (high-order pregnancy) are faced with the difficult options of continuing the pregnancy with all the risks previously described, terminating the entire pregnancy, or reducing the number of fetuses (multi-fetal pregnancy reduction – MFPR) in an effort to decrease the risk of maternal and fetal problems. MFPR is a specialized procedure done in the 1st trimester or early 2nd trimester, by high-risk pregnancy (maternal-fetal medicine) specialists to decrease the risks associated with preterm delivery. It is a procedure that can also create profound ethical dilemmas. The main risk of MFPR is loss of the entire pregnancy (about 1%, but can vary depending on doctor experience and number of fetuses present). Patients may opt to have the fetuses tested for genetic abnormalities before MFPR is performed.

Given these risks, it is important for you to work with your fertility team towards optimizing your chances for a singleton pregnancy. The following are strategies to consider:

1. If undergoing IVF, consider limiting the number of embryos to transfer. Ask your doctor about the ASRM embryo transfer guidelines and consider transferring a single day 5 embryo.
2. Consider using preimplantation genetic screening (PGS) to screen your embryos for genetic abnormalities and subsequently transfer a single, normal embryo.

3. If doing an intrauterine insemination (IUI) cycle, consider cancelling your cycle if more than two large follicles are present on day of hCG administration.
4. Prefer use of clomiphene or letrazole in conjunction with IUI cycles (instead of using gonadotropins).
5. If gonadotropins are used, ask about starting on a low dose (37.5 to 75 IU).

Quotes

"Just like others, I have found it hard to relax. I never sleep the night before the next ultrasound and worry when the babies don't move (which is a lot). I guess it just comes with the territory. Even though I haven't bled since 6 weeks 5 days, I still check the toilet paper every time I wipe!"

•••

"The one thing I've tried to do though is to be thankful for every day that I am pregnant and to try to enjoy watching myself "grow" and change. I LOVE the few times when I can feel the babies move and I try to focus on the fact that so far...things have gone well."

•••

"We are so excited...praying for twins! This was our last round of treatment ... so 2 for 1 would be great!"

•••

"Well my betas were high because it is twins. We had an ultrasound and it is two babies. I was so worried because the RE said my hCG numbers were really high. I know it sounds crazy but I am relieved it is only two. The RE scared me with discussing the possibility of selective reduction if more than two babies. We were blessed and it is twins!"

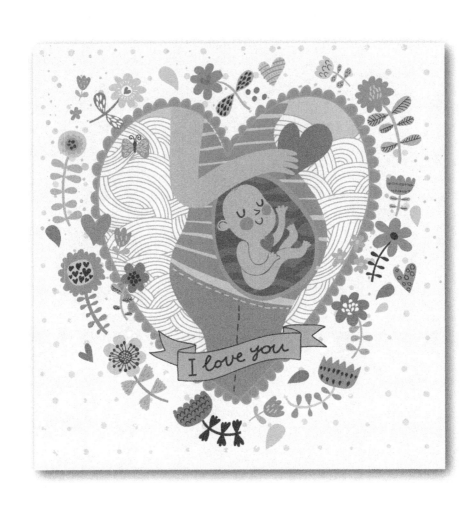

I love you

CHAPTER 47

Baby!

"Happiness does not depend on what happens outside of you,
but on what happens inside of you."
- Harold B. Lee

THERE IS PERHAPS no greater joy than putting all your sweat and tears into an effort that ultimately leads to the creation of a new life. Furthermore, this life is not just any life ... it originated from within you as a direct result of your love and effort.

Every human being should have the choice and ability to have a child. Fortunately, with our current medical tools and technology, every person now has this opportunity. The journey may not be easy or straightforward. However, the beauty and rewards that follow a successful pregnancy are remarkable and indescribable.

Know that there are millions of other women and men like you who are struggling to have a child. With the proper guidance and care, you will soon be one of the millions who now have the privilege of raising a beautiful child in this amazing world.

Tips

1. Send pictures of your baby to your fertility team. Better yet, stop by and see them with your baby. They will LOVE it!
2. Your fertility team will likely contact you to find out the outcome of your pregnancy. They need to collect this data to report their outcomes to the Centers for Disease Control & Prevention (CDC).

3. If you have frozen embryos and plan to have another child, talk to your fertility team a few months prior to when you plan to use them. They can guide you in planning early for a frozen embryo transfer.

4. If you have frozen embryos and no longer plan to have more children, consider donating your embryos to another couple struggling with infertility. Many fertility centers have an embryo donation program.

Quotes

"This infertility roller coaster definitely sucks. It took us absolutely forever, but we did eventually get our miracle. I'm certain yours is waiting for you -- and hopefully very soon!"

• • •

"Once the baby is born a whole new set of worries set in ... LOL. The most wonderful and scary thing ever!"

Part Eight

Extra

CHAPTER 48

Things Infertility Couples Do Not Want To Hear

1. Just Relax!
2. You're too stressed.
3. It's all in your head.
4. Why did you wait so long?
5. You're young … it will happen.
6. Be grateful you already have one child.
7. Maybe this is God's way of saying that it's not meant to be.
8. You're trying too hard.
9. You're not trying hard enough.
10. You just have to really want it.
11. As soon as you just stop trying, it will happen.
12. It will happen when the time is right.
13. God has a plan.
14. When are you going to have kids?
15. He's not shooting blanks is he?
16. All he has to do is look at me and I get pregnant.
17. You must be doing something wrong.
18. If it's meant to be, it will happen.
19. Go on vacation … that's how we had our kids.
20. We have four kids … you can gladly take one of ours.
21. You can always adopt.
22. Are you pregnant?

23. Do you have children?
24. You don't want kids … they keep you up all night.
25. It must be nice not to worry about birth control.
26. I told you that you were too into your career.
27. When you are pregnant, you'll have to …
28. You need to get healthy first.
29. At least it's fun trying!
30. You are single … why do you want to be tied down with kids?
31. Have you tried Chinese medicine?
32. Want to babysit?
33. Can you host my baby shower?
34. At least you get to sleep in.
35. I told you this would happen.
36. Guess what … I'm pregnant!

CHAPTER 49

Things Infertility Couples Do Want To Hear

1. Congratulations! You are pregnant!
2. It is not your fault.
3. Many couples have the same problem.
4. We can help finance your treatment.
5. Your chance of getting pregnant is excellent.
6. Your actions did not contribute to the miscarriage.
7. Even after several miscarriages, most couples go on to have a baby.
8. Tell me what you need … I am here to help.
9. Once you see a heartbeat on ultrasound, the chance of miscarriage drops significantly.
10. You are not alone.
11. We can start treatment right away.
12. I have many patients with similar issues who had success.
13. We can overcome this together.
14. I have the same problem.
15. Come with me to my support group … it really helps.
16. Stress is common and normal during this process.
17. It is okay to take a break if you need it.
18. I also went thru similar fertility treatments.
19. I know a great fertility doctor who can help you.
20. I will cover for you at work if you need time off.
21. We can provide sample medications to help with the cost.
22. Call me anytime if you need to talk.

23. Let's take a break and go on vacation.
24. Your insurance covers your fertility treatments!
25. It is okay to establish a career before starting your family.
26. You can freeze your eggs if you are not ready to have kids now.
27. Problems with sperm quality are very common and can be overcome.
28. I am sorry you are going thru so much stress.
29. You are doing everything you can.
30. Hang in there!
31. I love you no matter what happens.

References

Building Your Family. 2016 Infertility and Adoption Guide. New York: New Hope Media LLC. 2016.

Diamond MP, Legro RS, Coutifaris C, et al. Letrozole, Gonadotropin, or Clomiphene for Unexplained Infertility. N Engl J Med 2015;373:1230-1240.

Ethics Committee of ASRM. Consideration of the gestational carrier: a committee opinion. Fertil Steril 2013;99:1838-41.

Ethics Committee of ASRM. Disparities in access to effective treatment for infertility in the United States: an Ethics Committee opinion. Fertil Steril 2015;104:1104-10.

Legro RS, Barnhart HX, Schlaff WD, et al. Clomiphene, Metformin, or Both for Infertility in the Polycystic Ovary Syndrome. N Engl J Med 2007;356:551-566.

Legro RS, Brzyski RG, Diamond MP, et al. Letrozole versus Clomiphene for Infertility in the Polycystic Ovary Syndrome. N Engl J Med 2014;371:119-129.

Practice Committee of ACOG and ASRM. Female age-related fertility decline. Fertil Steril 2014;101:633-4.

References

Practice Committee of ASRM and SART. Optimizing natural fertility: a committee opinion. Fertil Steril 2013;100:631-7.

Practice Committee of ASRM and SART. Recommendations for practices utilizing gestational carriers: a committee opinion. Fertil Steril 2015;103:e1-8.

Practice Committee of ASRM and SART. Recommendations for gamete and embryo donation: a committee opinion. Fertil Steril 2013;99:47-62.

Schattman GL. Cryopreservation of Oocytes. N Engl J Med 2015;373:1755-60.

Appendix

Pertinent publications by Tarun Jain, MD:

- **Jain T**, Harlow BL, Hornstein MD. Insurance coverage and outcomes of in vitro fertilization. <u>N Engl J Med</u> 2002;347:661-6.
  **Accompanying Editorial: Guzick DS. Should insurance coverage be mandated. <u>N Engl J Med</u> 2002;347:686-8.

- **Jain T**, Klein NA, Lee DM, Sluss PM, Soules MR. Endocrine assessment of relative reproductive age in normal eumenorrheic younger and older women across multiple cycles. <u>Am J Obstet Gynecol</u> 2003;189:1080-4.

- **Jain T**, Hornstein MD. To pay or not to pay. <u>Fertil Steril</u> 2003;80:27-9.

- **Jain T**, Missmer SA, Hornstein MD. Trends in embryo-transfer practice and in outcomes of the use of assisted reproductive technology in the United States. <u>N Engl J Med</u> 2004;350:1639-45.
  ** Accompanying Editorial: Rebar RW, DeCherney AH. Assisted reproductive technology in the United States. <u>N Engl J Med</u> 2004;350:1603-4.

- **Jain T**, Soules MR, Collins JA. Comparison of basal follicle stimulating hormone versus the clomiphene citrate challenge test for ovarian reserve screening. <u>Fertil Steril</u> 2004;82:180-5.

Appendix

- **Jain T**, Missmer SA, Gupta RS, Hornstein MD. Pre-implantation sex selection demand and preferences in an infertility population. <u>Fertil Steril</u> 2005;83:649-58.

- **Jain T**, Barbieri RL. Website quality assessment: mistaking apples for oranges. <u>Fertil Steril</u> 2005;83:546-8.

- **Jain T**, Missmer SA, Hornstein MD. Trends in embryo-transfer practice and in outcomes of the use of assisted reproductive technology in the United States. <u>Obstet Gynecol Surv</u> 2005;60:176-78.

- **Jain T**, Hornstein MD. Disparities in access to infertility services in a state with mandated insurance coverage. <u>Fertil Steril</u> 2005;84:221-3.

- Dahl E, Gupta RS, Beutel M, Stoebel-Richter Y, Brosig B, Tinneberg H, **Jain T**. Pre-conception sex selection demand and preferences in the United States. <u>Fertil Steril</u> 2006;85:468-73.

- **Jain T**. Socioeconomic and racial disparities among infertility patients seeking care. <u>Fertil Steril</u> 2006;85:876-81.

- Abusef M, Hornstein MD, **Jain T**. Assessment of United States fertility clinic websites according to ASRM/SART guidelines. <u>Fertil Steril</u> 2007;87:88-92.

- Zaidi N, Scoccia B, Leach RL, **Jain T**. Moderate conscious sedation for in vitro fertilization oocyte retrieval procedures in an office setting. <u>Int J Anesth</u> 2007;12(1).

- **Jain T**, Gupta RS. Trends in utilization of intracytoplasmic sperm injection in the United States. <u>N Engl J Med</u> 2007;357:251-7.

- Stern JE, Cedars M, **Jain T**, Klein NA, Beaird M, Grainger D, Gibbons W. Assisted reproductive technology practice patterns and the impact of embryo transfer guidelines in the United States. <u>Fertil Steril</u> 2007;88:275-82.

- Gibbons W, Grainger D, Cedars M, **Jain T**, Klein N, Stern JE. Continuous quality improvement and assisted reproductive technology multiple gestations: some progress, some answers, more questions. <u>Fertil Steril</u> 2007;88:301-4.

- **Jain T**, Gupta RS. Increased use of ICSI for treatment of infertility other than male-factor infertility. <u>Nature Clin Pract Urology</u> 2007;4:579-80.

- Missmer SA, **Jain T**. Sex selection demand and preferences among infertility patients in Midwestern United States. <u>J Assist Reprod Genet</u> 2007;24:451-7.

- **Jain T**, Missmer SA. Support for selling embryos among infertility patients. <u>Fertil Steril</u> 2008;90:564-8.

- **Jain T**, Missmer SA. Support for embryonic stem cell research among infertility patients. <u>Fertil Steril</u> 2008;90:506-12.

- **Jain T**, Luke B, Leach RE. Assisted reproductive technology and perinatal outcomes: What you and your patients should know. <u>ACOG Update</u> September, 2008.

- Abusef M, Missmer SA, Barbieri RL, **Jain T**, Hornstein MD. Geographic distribution of Reproductive Endocrinology and Infertility (REI) fellowships in the United States. <u>Fertil Steril</u> 2009;91:1636-41.

- Fujimoto VY, Luke B, Brown MB, **Jain T**, Armstrong A, Grainger DA, Hornstein MD. Racial and ethnic disparities in assisted reproductive technology (ART) outcomes in the United States. <u>Fertil Steril</u> 2010;93:382-90.

Appendix

- Fujimoto V, **Jain T**, Alvero R, Nelson LM, Catherino WH, Olatinwo M, Marsh EE, Broomfield D, Taylor H, Armstrong AY. Proceedings from the conference on reproductive problems in women of color. Fertil Steril 2010;94:7-10.

- Missmer SA, Seifer DB, **Jain T**. Cultural factors contributing to health care disparities among patients with infertility in Midwestern United States. Fertil Steril 2011;95:1943-9.

- Seifer DB, Sharara FI, **Jain T** (2013). Toward a Better Understanding of Racial Disparities in Utilization and Outcomes of IVF Treatment in the USA. In F.I. Sharara (Ed.), *Ethnic Differences in Fertility and Assisted Reproduction* (pp. 239-44). New York, NY: Springer.

Appendix

Resources

A. Reproductive Medicine Organizations
  1. American Society for Reproductive Medicine - ASRM (www.asrm.org)
  2. American College of Obstetrics & Gynecology - ACOG (www.acog.org)
  3. Society for Assisted Reproductive Technology - SART (www.sart.org)
  4. The Society of Reproductive Surgeons - SRS (www.reprodsurgery.org)
  5. Society for Male Reproduction & Urology – SMRU (www.smru.org)
  6. American Academy of Assisted Reproductive Technology Attorneys (www.aarta.org)

B. Advocacy / Support Groups
  1. RESOLVE: The National Infertility Association (www.resolve.org)
  2. Fertility Within Reach (www.fertilitywithinreach.org)
  3. Fertile Hope (www.livestrong.org/fertilehope)
  4. Frank Talk (www.franktalk.org)
  5. Choice Moms (www.choicemoms.org)

C. Online medical information
  1. Reproductive Facts - ASRM (www.reproductivefacts.org)
  2. Office of Women's Health – US Department of Health (www.womenshealth.gov)
  3. Merck Manual (www.merckmanual.com/home)
  4. MedlinePlus – US National Library of Medicine (www.nlm.nih.gov/medlineplus)
  5. Healthy Women (www.healthywomen.org)